Eyes Without Sparkle

A journey through postnatal illness

Elaine A Hanzak

Forewords by

Diana Lynn Barnes
and
Judith Ellis

To Jane,

Let's keep helping others to sparkle!

Best wishes,

Elaine Hanzak.

Radcliffe Publishing
Oxford • Seattle

Radcliffe Publishing Ltd
18 Marcham Road
Abingdon
Oxon OX14 1AA
United Kingdom

www.radcliffe-oxford.com
Electronic catalogue and worldwide online ordering facility.

British Library Cataloguing in Publication Data

A catalogue record for this book is available from the British Library.

ISBN 1 85775 655 X

Typeset by Acorn Bookwork Ltd, Salisbury, Wiltshire
Printed and bound by TJ International Ltd, Padstow, Cornwall

To my 'boys' Nick and Dominic.
Without you two there would be no story.
With you there will always be the deepest of love and devotion
. . . and very sparkly eyes!

Contents

Foreword

Most women who have known the profound experience of pregnancy and childbirth have a story to tell. For some, it's the story about the rigors of long labor or the disruption in daily life caused by morning sickness throughout pregnancy. For others, it's an account of their excitement the moment they discovered, after months of trying for a baby, that they had finally conceived. But the story we've all heard, whether or not we've given birth, is the one that depicts pregnancy as glorious and new motherhood as a time of uncontainable euphoria and ultimate fulfillment as two becomes three and a family is born. It's this narrative that has become a part of our oral tradition – a story handed down from generation to generation.

Yet, in the shadows of these cultural myths that romanticize the transition between pregnancy and motherhood lurks a different story. It is one that rarely gets told because the women in these stories sit too often in silence, filled with shame and self-recrimination because they believe somehow that their own actions have caused this seemingly unexplainable revolt against their psyche.

With great courage, Elaine Hanzak shares the story of her battle with a rare, but potentially life-threatening illness called postpartum psychosis, describing in intimate detail the unraveling of her mind as she struggled to maintain sanity in the face of this illness that knows no boundaries and makes no distinctions between realities. She has eloquently used her own experience to educate and inform the professional community about mental illness while at the same time providing women and their families with the tools to advocate for their own medical and emotional care.

Because Elaine knew of my work as the president of Postpartum Support International and my involvement as a psychotherapist who treats women with depression and other mood disorders that occur during pregnancy and in the postpartum period, she asked me, earlier this year, if I would review her unfinished manuscript. At the time she did not know that, in addition to my clinical work in this field, I too had known the horrors of a severe postpartum depression after the birth of my precious daughter, my second child, almost thirteen years ago. It was a depression that lingered ferociously for three years due to the lack of medical knowledge about postpartum mood disorders and the subsequent ineffective treatments I received. And so, I resonate, both personally and professionally with Elaine's story and I applaud her willingness to share her own experience in the hope of increasing public awareness about these insidious illnesses that occur around childbearing.

Every day I treat competent, responsible women, women like Elaine Hanzak. They are women who lead fulfilling lives, with loving partners and supportive families; unexpectedly they find their normal lives shaken by this illness that can creep in gradually or strike suddenly without warning. Postpartum depression and postpartum psychosis cross the lines of age, culture, ethnicity and socioeconomic status. They can lead to the fragmentation of a woman's energy and spirit at a time in her life when she is most in need of physical and emotional stamina. It can interfere in the blossoming attachment relationship between a mother and her infant with potentially long range repercussions for the healthy social, emotional and cognitive development of that child. It can wreak havoc as the entire family attempts to cope with the stress brought on by the demands of a new baby and the debilitation of a new mother's depression.

Using her story as the framework, Elaine highlights the symptoms of depression and psychosis that women go through during the course of these illnesses. She tells of the suicidal thoughts, the volatility, the restlessness and agitation. She reveals the pain in feeling emotionally detached from her child whose birth was the fulfillment of her dreams. We hear about the barrage of intruding thoughts that beckoned her to harm her own child, the images of self-injury and her horror at these alien thoughts as she struggled to maintain normalcy in the midst of emotional and psychological chaos.

Elaine Hanzak's story is a story of hope and determination, opening the door to the reader's deeper understanding of the complexities of this illness as it affects all women who battle them and the 'roller coaster ride of emotions,' as she describes it. Her story underscores the false beliefs that circulate around pregnancy and childbirth. It's these romantic ideals that pit societal expectations against the stark reality that the months following delivery are anything *but* peaceful for most new mothers.

As Elaine herself discovered through the progression of her psychosis and her own recovery, postpartum illness is not the result of a character flaw or a personality defect. Our societal notions that 'strong' people are not vulnerable to depression leave too many women embarrassed by the feelings they are having, afraid of being judged as weak or bad, and even fearful that their baby could be taken away. The stigmas attached to mental illness interfere with accurate assessment, recognition of the problem, and proper treatment.

Although postpartum psychosis may be rare, mood changes around pregnancy and childbirth are not. As many as four out of five women who give birth will experience some minor change in their mental health following the delivery of their child. Of those women, 10–15% will come to know the challenges of postpartum depression. Thank you, Elaine for speaking out in the hope that your own very moving story will change the tide of thinking about perinatal mood disorders and improve women's healthcare experiences at such a pivotal time in their lives.

Diana Lynn Barnes, PsyD MFT
President Postpartum Support International (2002–2004)
The Center for Postpartum Health, California
November 2004

Foreword

On each encounter with the health service a patient brings a story, not only of their current problem or need, but a story of the journey they have taken to reach this point, this encounter, often with the final destination still unknown. In the busy climate of a healthcare setting, where patients are insecure and unsure and staff appear busy and focused upon the here and now, these stories are seldom sought or shared. Yet, without the story little sense can be made of the present. Care can only be planned to meet perceived needs and, therefore, in its delivery, care may well not meet the actual needs of the individual.

Everyone's journey is different, bringing something unique to each encounter but, like pieces of a jigsaw, may look the same but slot into a different position. In the same way a patient's diagnosis is likely to have been encountered before by professionals and, therefore, professionals can provide well-meaning reassurances of normal progress. These are, however, difficult to accept in relation to the whole picture, what we view as our own unique circumstances. This is where patient and indeed carer support groups are of so much importance, reassuring that someone 'really' understands how the journey feels and can be there beside and in support. However, for each of us this is our own journey. This book describes Elaine's journey. It is an honest and moving account that takes us from an existence many can identify with or seek, a happy family life with the joy of childbirth ahead, into a world that we hope personally never to enter but which for some, including those around us or cared for by us, is all too recognisable and real.

I met Elaine for the first time in 1999 as she was living the final chapters of this book – it was the same day she was to go on and meet Lionel Richie! Elaine had been asked to tell us her story with a particular focus upon fundamental aspects of care that had affected the quality of her varied experience of the health service as a patient, mother and daughter. Elaine's talk, accompanied by a series of family photos such as you would find in any album, was stunningly powerful, generating in the audience reflection on the effectiveness of their own practice, specifically in getting the basics right.

At the conclusion of the conference Elaine was inundated with requests to share her story which reinforced her already strong motivation to write about her experiences, her journey.

For professionals this book provides not only a powerful story but a trigger for reflection. It reinforces the need for healthcare staff to consider the complete patient journey and the effect each event may have upon later experiences and interpretation. It also highlights the importance of caring and compassion, and the 'little things' in getting the quality of patient experience right. The inclusive gesture, kind word and act are movingly described as supporting and aiding recovery and, to the contrary, the devastating short- and long-term effects of thoughtless comments and uncaring dismissal are shared.

In the NHS Plan published in July 2000[1] health service staff are expected to listen and hear patients. It is fundamental for quality healthcare. Health service staff have to listen, not just to 'expert patients',[2] who have learnt to express their stories and needs in terms staff understand and feel comfortable with, but to all in need of their involvement. From the first encounter, making sense of information given must include wariness and acceptance of what has been left unsaid. Without the whole picture, people's reactions or fears may be unfathomable. However, the picture may be difficult to build. Information may not be freely shared, cast aside by either patient or professional as irrelevant, too private or potentially threatening. There requires recognition by all, including carers and families that nothing is irrelevant or must be too readily dismissed from consideration. Completing the picture, understanding the journey that patient, family and carers have taken, will support a partnership in planning and action that will ensure care can meet the actual, not merely the professionally perceived needs of individuals. Elaine's story above all reinforces that, however busy, however complex, for a quality patient experience the journey has to be shared.

Judith Ellis MBE, PhD, MSc, BSc(Hons), PGCE
Chief Nurse and Director of Workforce Development
Great Ormond Street Hospital
November 2004

References

1 Department of Health (2000) The National Health Service Plan for England: A plan for investment a plan for reform. DoH, London.
2 Department of Health (2004) The Expert Patient: A new approach to chronic disease management for the 21st century. DoH, London.

Acknowledgements

Although at times my illness made me feel isolated and alone I am well aware and very appreciative of all those who played a part in my recovery. I definitely was not on my own!

If I had not become a mother this book would never have been written, and many of the events described would not have happened. Although it has been a saga, the final product is our delightful son, Dominic. He brings me joy, pride and a maternal glow which are undoubtedly worth all the struggles. Thank you Dominic for being you and wanting to share our story with others because you want it to help them. Thank you also for the wonderful design you did for the cover of our book, which you created early one holiday morning before we all got up.

My darling husband Nick has been my rock and my support throughout. He is a much more private person than me and I am grateful for his willingness to share the many intimate details of our life together with you, the reader. I cherish our times together and look forward to many, many more years of 'us'.

My parents have been a support at every step of the way, from making Sunday meals to sharing my passion for certain music! Knowing how it feels to see your child suffer, it cannot have been easy for either of them over these last few years, especially as a person with a mental illness can be so hard to help. Yet their love and support has been a significant factor on my road back to full health. Nick's mother has also been an asset and support to us all. In reading the original manuscript of this book they were all amazed at what actually happened and had not realised at the time as I was so good at hiding the truth. Additional thanks go to my mother for the hours she spent checking the Appendix details.

Big brother Kevin and his family plus 'little sis' Claire have also helped along the way and must have felt 'pushed out' at times by my needs. Although we were separated by distance during these years, I always knew I was in your thoughts and help was there when I needed it. Likewise with my sister-in-law Glenys and her son Patrick.

My grandparents were often a 'port in a storm' and always would put the kettle on! I know I was able to help them with their hospital visits and daily tasks but in doing so, that helped me. It is a pity that my Grandma is now not fully able to comprehend that our family stories are to be published, but she smiles sweetly as I tell her. I know Grandpa would have said, 'That's grand, love!' The staff at Halton Haven, where he died, were wonderful with us all.

Friendships can be truly tested at times of ill health. Many people do not understand mental illness and can be very judgemental and critical. I was lucky with the love and support, both emotional and practical, from the two Sues and their families. Their friendship extended beyond the call of duty on many occasions, and continues to do so. My battles would have been much worse without you two and for that I shall remain forever grateful.

Other friends and neighbours who have also been an encouragement to us include Margaret and Richard, Carol and Ian, Diane and Jon, Roy and Beverley, Carole and Catherine, Janet and Kevin, Debbie and Alan, Jenny, Diane, Richard, Jeannie, Margaret and Jeanette.

I know my absence at work caused problems for many people and I appreciate the efforts which had to be made to overcome them. My colleagues, pupils and their parents at school have been supportive, with fond memories of those who are no longer with us – Dorothy, Charlotte, John and Dale. The therapists and medical staff at school have been particularly helpful in their encouragement over the years – thank you, Gwen and Karen.

Of course I am very appreciative of the good aspects of the nursing, medical and other staff involved in my treatment and care. My general practitioner, health visitor and community psychiatric nurse were all particularly helpful, and I shall never, ever forget the wonderful nurse who wrapped me in a blanket and gave me a milky drink after I had been attacking her!

I would also like to thank the midwifery team who brought Dominic into the world, especially Helen and the anonymous lady at my side! Also the excellent paediatric teams who nursed him at later stages, particularly Glynis. Cathy and her family, who looked after Dominic as a toddler, were another strong help to us all.

The members of the groups I attended whilst Dominic was small also helped to play their parts – National Childbirth Trust members; antenatal class; Mums and Tots; Ray and Anne Samuels plus members of their congregation.

I am also grateful to members of the general public who have helped me either practically, e.g. with folding a pram, or by simply admiring Dominic; small gestures but they meant a great deal to me at the time. In a similar way, helpful staff in pubs, restaurants and shops. Never underestimate a little act or expression of kindness to a mentally ill person or new mother, in particular, as it can often make or break their day. Daytime television can also have the same effect!

Several people have been great motivators in me actually compiling and getting this book into print. I must thank Margi for asking me to give my first talk and then Mandie for inviting me to do the London talk. Of course I am eternally grateful to Peggie Ward for giving me the skills and confidence to speak in public. Flo Longhorn, was a source of encouragement too; when at times I was faltering and felt I was wasting my time she renewed my self-confidence. I must thank Lindsey for interviewing me for her dissertation as her transcript helped me recall many events and feelings. My new friend Sam motivated me, on the beach in Mallorca, to begin the publishing journey and subsequently my friends Lyndsey, Ian and Sarah for making sure I did not give up. From then I have been grateful to Carolyn Scott, Editor of the journal *Professional Nurse*, for her publishing support and encouragement. There are several health professionals whom I would like to specifically thank with respect to completion of my book, particularly as I know how busy they all are with their particular roles. I wish to thank Sarah Mullally, Chief Nursing Officer, for writing a wonderful review and giving her permission to include quotes from it, on the back cover in particular. Likewise to Alex Vjestica, nursing lecturer and Stuart Clarke, Assistant Director for Psychological Therapies, Brooker Centre, Runcorn.

I am very grateful to Judith Ellis, Chief Nurse and Director of Workforce Development at Great Ormond Street, for encouraging me to persevere and complete this book and then for giving it her stamp of approval with a terrific review and foreword. We must have another early morning swim sometime!

I was delighted when Diana Lynn Barnes, President of Postpartum Support International and The Center for Postpartum Health in California, offered to write a foreword to the book. I was thrilled that she was able to give it her personal endorsement and recognise my journey as being relevant at an international level.

Also to Thelma Osborn, Health Visitor and Counsellor specialising in postnatal depression, for adding her chapter which puts my personal experience into a wider perspective of the illness and for others to reflect upon in their treatment of other patients.

My gratitude to Lionel Richie, for I know his inspiring music will always be there for me and make me want to 'dance on the ceiling'!

Thank you Gillian Nineham for believing that my story was worth sharing and Mike Mahoney for making me believe in myself again in more recent times (but that's another story!).

Thank you to everyone for bearing with me through the ups and downs of my life in recent years!

Finally, to the lady who inspired me to write a book about my illness 'as it would help so many people', here it is – I hope I have not disappointed you.

Introduction

In November 2000 I was the keynote speaker at a conference called 'Making a Difference in Patient Care', jointly organised by the National Health Service Executive and the journal *Professional Nurse*. I spoke about 'what matters to patients' and based it upon my personal experiences. Four years earlier I had been on the brink of a breakdown due to postnatal illness and a build-up in the variety of stresses of modern-day living. Since then I have recovered sufficiently to return to my full-time teaching career and lead a fulfilling life again.

Although my illness was due to postnatal problems, my symptoms, treatment and the effect upon my life have shown to be very similar to those faced by other people with different conditions. I have been surprised by the parallels with those, for example, who have other mental illnesses, who may have been bereaved and indeed with anyone who has needed a stay in a hospital bed. The fundamental needs of patients are the same regardless of diagnosis.

The strategies which were successful in helping me to recover are a personal reflection and I appreciate that they may not be useful to everyone. I am grateful to be well again and to be a stronger person after such a humbling experience of being 'totally out of control'.

Many people who heard my conference talk, and at other occasions, encouraged me to fully recall the events of this era of my life. In doing so, I would like professionals involved in nursing and treating patients to realise how their actions, good and bad, can have considerable implications upon a person's recovery. I also wish to inspire others by my story, who may be suffering in ways similar to me, and to give them, and their families and friends, hope, confidence and the will to carry on.

One day you *will* feel better.

Elaine A Hanzak
November 2004

Prologue

Sandwiched between a bedside cabinet and a wardrobe, I sat rhythmically banging my head against the wall. I was gouging holes out of my own increasingly bloody hands and fingers using my nails. I was in a dimly lit psychiatric ward in the building of a former Victorian asylum. It was almost Christmas Eve and the other patients were asleep, some snoring, some fidgeting, but none seemed peaceful in mind or body. I was too scared to ask for help to soothe the involuntary body jerks which wracked my whole being. The previous night I had been severely reprimanded by a nurse for being a 'troublemaker' and I knew she was on duty again.

What was I doing in here? I was a sensible 33-year-old mother of a beautiful baby boy. I had a loving husband, a supportive family. I had a career I loved as a school teacher. I had a comfortable home and lifestyle. I even had two handsome cats! To most people I had 'everything', so why was I now a shadow of my former self? A broken, useless woman who was too frightened to ask for help from those who should have been able to help.

How did I get here . . . and would I ever get out?

CHAPTER 1

My life before becoming a 'Hanzak'

'Children bring their love,' said my dying grandmother, as she patted my mother's bump (me!). Unfortunately she did not live long enough to actually meet me. Yet I shared her belief about children for many years, until illness proved the theory wrong, for a while. My middle name, Anne, was chosen after that special lady.

I was the second child of Lawrence and Maureen Walsh, born at a maternity home in Fleetwood, Lancashire on Sunday 4 August, 1963. My elder brother Kevin, who was two when I was born, had been a perfect baby who slept, ate and charmed everyone to the book. I did not! My sleep pattern was terrible but my worst problem was crying constantly until I was picked up. Sometimes if a woman tried to calm me it did not work, but put me in a man's arms and I was happy. I have never changed! My parents tried everything to soothe me and eventually they were told by a doctor that all I needed was to feel loved and secure and not to worry.

'All children are different,' he reassured them.

My mother, an only child, had trained as an assistant librarian and my father left school at 15 to join the Royal Air Force. He was from a large family in Greenock, Scotland. They had met in Blackpool, whilst my father was based in Lancashire, and settled in nearby Thornton Cleveleys. It was rare in the 1960s for families to 'move away'. Our small town was a typical 'retirement' area, whose residents often felt their aspirations lay higher than those associated with the brashness of Blackpool, and compared to the austere 1940s and 1950s, our standard of living was high. It was generally a time of hope, progress, community involvement, care and safety. It was a time and place when aspirations could become real – and did. Both my parents had wanted their own children and although we were not wealthy, we were rich in the attention, love and interest they bestowed on us. I always wanted a family like ours when I grew up. My chosen childhood books described the classic family with a boy and a girl; a mother who stayed at home and a father who went out to work. My parents had the typical problems of coping with shift-work, limited wages, each other and a young family, but to me we resembled the epitome of a happy life. My dreams of having this for myself one day were normal at the time and many of the modern-day stresses did not exist then, especially the notion of being a 'working' mother.

My childhood years were fulfilling and I was contented. My father worked shifts on jobs usually involved in fire-fighting and safety whilst my mother stayed at home to care for us. We lived in a small, three-bedroomed, semi-detached house. Kevin and I would often play happily together and we participated in many after-school activities. I was busy with Brownies, then Guides; dancing classes for ballet and tap; Sunday school and playing the cello. We would play family games some evenings and often had days out at the weekend with my maternal grandparents, who had a car. From an early age I learnt to be busy and enjoyed being so, although there was never any pressure to attend these activities. The years ticked by with happy memories of school, playing out with the local children, shopping and meals at my grandparents, in nearby Fleetwood, every Friday night. We would have an annual holiday, usually to a caravan on a farm or boating on the Norfolk Broads. At school I was usually quite successful but had to work reasonably hard to achieve 'B' grades. Kevin seemed to find academic skills easy and managed 'A' grades with apparently little effort.

Right from being able to walk and talk I adored children. I was the classic little girl who wanted dolls' prams and to play 'house'. My grandmother often used to come and play and we would spend hours with me being 'Mummy' to my dolls and acting out events such as christenings in my bedroom. We always used to have lovely birthday parties. My father was great at entertaining children and making us feel special. However, I always used to say to my parents that I would have no Christmas presents and no birthday presents ever again, if only I could have a baby brother or sister. When I was ten we moved to a slightly larger house in Fleetwood; I also got the dreamed-of little sister and I have had presents ever since too! At the time many people commented to my parents that she 'must have been a shock'. They were annoyed as she was actually planned. So at ten years old I had the nearest thing to my own little baby, a sister named Claire. I idolised her. I did everything for her – I bathed her, fed her and changed her. We shared a bedroom. She was my little living doll. I took delight in all her stages of development and she fed my hunger even more to be a mother in the years to come.

The decision to move was mainly to be near the local grammar school, which had an excellent reputation. Our new home overlooked its playing fields. Fleetwood is a fishing port but its industry was in decline at this time. My grandparents were delighted that we moved within a mile from them but my parents had the foresight to realise that their own children's future would lie outside this area, and good education would be the passport to success. I always remember my mother and father being supportive in all our childhood activities. I admire them for making sure we got the opportunities they did not have. They gave us a great deal of time, effort and everything they could provide. This is reflected in the fact my brother has spent his career learning and teaching in universities worldwide and my younger sister has got both a Masters plus a first-class Honours degree.

My younger teens were very involved with Claire. This was not to the exclusion of the usual teenage things, but as opposed to watching television I would rather be playing games with her. One favourite game was to make a den between our beds. I had some best friends and was mad about all boys from the age of about 13 – just a typical teenager really. My later teens were busily spent on homework, Claire and the standard infatuation with a boy who lived across the road. I never rebelled and never went through any wild phases. I suppose I was boring. My reports always said I was mature and sensible. How I hated that description! My best friend at the time was very attractive and won local beauty competitions. Most of the time, I must admit as a teenager, I felt very much under her shadow as she had a beautiful face and figure. I always felt that if a boy showed any interest in me it was because they wanted to get to know her better! Guess who the boy across the road asked out? Yes – it was her!

Meanwhile I began to wonder what my choice of career would be. I often used to read a book called *Careers for Girls* to help me. Soon I realised that I wanted to become a speech therapist. My parents had sent Kevin and me for elocution lessons, as it was considered to be a useful course during this era. I went for 11 years and loved it. My teacher, Peggie Ward, taught me the skills to speak in public and founded an interest in the English language that has remained with me. The older girls who went to elocution did their diploma in speech and language there and I always wanted to do it. I knew that it could lead to speech therapy and this became my ambition.

In the summer of 1978 I had just finished my 'O' levels and Kevin had taken his 'A' levels, when we all moved to Runcorn, in Cheshire, due to our father's promotion within ICI. At the time this was one of the UK's largest companies and promotion and moving around the country had become more commonplace. My maternal grandparents were devastated and reacted as though we were going to the other side of the world, not 70 miles away. To their generation you were born, worked, lived and died in the same area and did not desert your home town. In spite of their reservations we did move and all the family benefited. Our new home was roughly between Manchester and Liverpool. Runcorn has its roots in the chemical industry and from the building of the Jubilee Bridge across the River Mersey, it had become a designated 'new town', and was undergoing tremendous development in housing, transport and industry. Our house was on the edge of the 'old' town and we soon all settled in. Kevin and I had a great summer together as he had also just learnt to drive and we commandeered the family car. We both got holiday jobs and amused ourselves in the evenings by getting to know people locally. In the autumn Kevin went on to Oxford University and I went into the sixth form. I was surprised at that point that people actually talked to me and not just because I had a glamorous friend. I had several romances and I loved it! My only regret at leaving Fleetwood was that I had to leave my elocution lessons and consequently was not able to pursue the diploma.

During my final year at school I had my life mapped out. I wanted to go to university, be a speech therapist for a few years, be married at 24 and have a family by 28. I would definitely give up work for a while because at that time I did not agree with the philosophy of being a working mother. Why should you bring a child into this world if you could not look after it 24 hours a day? Yet it did not work out that way ultimately for me and many others. In the early 1980s there were still many mothers who stayed at home but since then it seems that Britain has had a major change in its values and society as most women now work and bring up a family too, adding to the stresses of modern-day living.

The week before I did my 'A' levels I was in a car crash with some friends, breaking my wrist and being very shaken. Consequently I did not do as well as I should have done in my exams. Whilst I had been researching speech therapy I had kept coming across the words 'mental handicap', and did not know anything about it. So during the sixth form I started helping at the local school for such children and loved it. My parents advised me that a teaching job for a mother is a great bonus, due to the holidays, and rather than resit my 'A' levels I decided upon this alternative career. It was a decision I generally do not regret. Four years later I qualified with an Honours degree in Education with a specialism for children with mental handicaps, or learning difficulties which is now more accurate. I studied at Edge Hill College, in Ormskirk, Lancashire and thoroughly enjoyed my time there. It was a quiet campus in a rural setting but the course and social life suited me. I made some good friends, some of whom I still see regularly. I had a steady boyfriend during my college years and for a while thought we may marry. However, once away from the campus we drifted apart, but I shall always treasure my special memories of that era.

Once qualified, I got a job teaching nursery children at a special school in Chester and was able to live with my parents again. As I did not have my own house to run, socially there was a big gap and I filled it with a group called 'Rotaract'. This is the junior version of Rotary International and is basically a club for 18–30 year-olds who organise social and fundraising events. I loved the planning and all the activities and was the president one year, when we raised about £5000 for local charities.

I had a happy and contented life around that time and I also met my first husband through the 'Rotaract' club. He was a solicitor and I thought he was everything I ever wanted. It was all slotting into place. We were married a week before my 25th birthday, just within a few days of my overall aim of being married at 24, and I thought that was it. Unfortunately, just after we were engaged, I was chatting about our future together and hopes for children when my fiancé said, 'To be honest I would not be fussed if we never had them.'

At this point I heard the warning bells of course and replied, 'Look, we need to sort this out, because I desperately want children. I admit not immediately, but I know it's something that I really do want.'

We tentatively agreed to wait five years.

Initially it felt like the perfect marriage and I appreciated all that our lifestyle provided. However, as the years went by we started having all sorts of problems, not just about the prospect of having a family of our own. As several of my peer group were having children, I was feeling more and more left out and the maternal ache became intense. Meanwhile my husband kept saying things like, 'Oh children, they ruin your life.'

Just after we had been married I had moved jobs back to the original special school where I had helped out as a sixth-form student. For a while I was the nursery teacher and thoroughly enjoyed working with disabled toddlers and their parents. After a few years I transferred to the leavers' unit for 16–19 year-old students. Our class base was in a self-contained bungalow on the playing field and our focus was on life skills. My assistant and I worked hard in encouraging the youngsters to achieve targets in all curriculum areas and we even had several students who went out on work experience placements. As my pupils' confidence increased, mine did too. One day we had a very useful staff training day concerning assertiveness. The main message that I picked up from it was that if you have a problem you have two alternatives. If you cannot do anything about the problem, why worry. Alternatively, if you are in a position to do something, then get on with it!

This made me realise that I had been pretending my marriage was fine for a long time and I faced the fact that I had grown apart from my husband. We both had to reluctantly acknowledge this and tried to solve our differences, but unsuccessfully. Just before I was 30 I moved back to my parents again, became divorced and threw myself into work.

CHAPTER 2

Nick and I

I had felt very stifled at times in my first marriage as my husband was caring but overly cautious about many things. My favourite song became 'Reckless and Impulsive' by Wilson Phillips. I bought myself a fast, sporty car, had my hair cut short (my ex-husband did not like it that way) and generally wanted to live life more adventurously. I met up with college and 'Rotaract' friends and organised many social events. For my 30th birthday we had an excellent summer barbecue at my parents, complete with bonfire and merriment into the early hours. My goal of having a child by 28 had faded like the flames did.

At school a teaching colleague, called Nick, and I became good friends. He was eight years older than me, had never married, and lived an active lifestyle. Together we began to go hiking, cycling and for meals out. We took some of our pupils to France on holiday together and our friendship blossomed. We even did a sponsored parachute jump for school and went skiing. How I enjoyed being reckless and impulsive! He was generous, kind and made me smile. The desire to be together grew stronger as our romance and love blossomed and in May 1994 we bought a house together in Runcorn, where we still live. The rate at which we transformed the house and garden amazed us. We both liked planning, choosing and buying our new decor and furnishings. Many hours were spent busily making the house our own and we often commented on what a good team we made. Both of us are very tidy and organised (some may say boringly so), but we like it!

Within a few months we began to plan our wedding and on 17 June 1995 we were married at the local registry office. Family and friends joined us for a buffet back at our house, and then some of us went on to a hotel on the outskirts of Chester for an intimate dinner. Nick and I stayed in a suite there for two nights, a short but blissful honeymoon. We chose this particular time, as opposed to school holidays, to coincide with my brother, his wife and new baby visiting England. He had met Annie, his wife, in her native Zimbabwe, where they still lived. Being a strong 'family-minded' girl, it would not have been as special if they had not been there.

Second time round, rule number one was that I wanted children and initially Nick was somewhat reluctant because he had lived on his own for 12 years. He was very much set in his ways, and as far as he was concerned he felt he was a bit too old for children. Years earlier he had presumed that he would have a family but after some unlucky relationships had given up on the idea. However, we had talked about it long and hard, and before we even got the house together we agreed that we would try for a family. I still felt very much that I wanted to be married before I had a baby. I am quite old-fashioned in that way, and very luckily, I was ecstatic as within three months of us being married, I was pregnant.

The baby was conceived on my 32nd birthday and I was over the moon. A couple of days after my birthday we went on a touring holiday in northern Spain with my parents to rural areas where pregnancy kits cannot be easily purchased! So we had to wait until our return to confirm it. I just knew I was pregnant. Normally I cannot keep any secrets from my mother as I either tell her or she guesses. I was dying to reveal my suspicions to her whilst we were away but managed not to. Afterwards she said she had realised I was expecting as my obvious silence on the subject of periods spoke volumes! In the previous two months I had commented on my disappointment. I remember lying in bed on my birthday just being aware that a miracle of nature was happening inside me – the miracle I had dreamed of all my life. It reminded me of my childhood plea to my parents. This was to be a birthday present I would never forget!

Yet the pregnancy path was not smooth. The first blow that fell was that we both had thought that maternity leave was on full pay but discovered the day after I had done the pregnancy test that this was not the case. At the time, we had spent a fortune on our house and the wedding and had tried to fit into 18 months what most couples take 15 years to do. Nick and I had decided that for financial reasons I would have to go back to work if we had a family. I liked my job, although given the choice I would have preferred not to work. I loved Nick deeply and felt content with him. He did more than me around the house and so I did not feel that I would have to do everything for a family. We both taught so would have the advantage of the school holidays with any children we may have. We lived close to our workplace and also would have some support from my parents and Nick's mother. I felt that I could manage being a working mother – so many people do, why couldn't I? I thrive on being busy so was convinced we would manage well.

If we had realised about the finances, we probably would have left trying for a baby a bit longer so that we could have cleared some of our debts and saved up a bit. However, we had not and I was determined that money worries would not cloud my delight at being an expectant mother. I wanted the whole world to know my condition and told the news to the rest of the family and friends almost immediately. On returning to work that September we had some training days. One of these involved lifting and handling techniques for people with special needs. The instructor asked if anyone had any particular physical problems or were pregnant, as they could not follow the practical aspects of the course. I admit to being extremely pleased to confess I was!

That pleasurable feeling extended across all areas of my life. Like most things I am ever involved in, I bought all the magazines and bought the books. When I had been getting married I had devoured the bridal magazines; when we bought the house I had delved into home-making journals. I did not feel I had an idyllic approach but I like looking into projects, researching them, finding out and making my own choices. Being pregnant was a wonderful venture for me. I began making lists of all the items we would need; sent off for mail-order catalogues by the dozen and researched every aspect of consumer advice into each maternity and baby product available. We decorated one of the two front bedrooms in a bright, primary-coloured scheme, hoping it would suit a boy or girl.

I was very, very excited about it. In addition, within the family, Nick has only got one sister, who had a single teenage son, so his mother had not had another new grandchild for years. My parents also only had one little grandson, Brendan, but at the time he lived in Africa and they did not see him very often. Consequently this baby would be the first grandchild they would be able to watch growing up day by day. All the family were excited and were looking forward to the baby coming. I continued to revel in the maternity clothes and decorating and furnishing the nursery. There was a slight financial worry but we knew once I got back to work it would solve the problem.

The first seven months of pregnancy I definitely bloomed. I was hardly sick, my hair and skin were shiny and the excitement of it all kept me very high in spirits. During the autumn term in school I tried to get ahead. I wanted to leave my class plus all the documentation in perfect order for my replacement and kept myself very busy. I loved being pregnant, especially at Christmas, and kept dreaming of the ones to come.

I began my first diary about the baby that January on a beautiful baby calendar full of gorgeous photographs and idyllic sayings. If I did anything related to the pregnancy I made a note of it. I began to knit a 'Golly' because as a child my favourite great auntie had always knitted me soft toys and I had vowed to do the same for any child of mine. I also was very excited that I could actually see my stomach moving and feel the baby kicking. 'Baby H', as we had christened our unborn child, definitely had a fidget after every evening meal and when I was ready to go to sleep. At my 24-week check-up the midwife said that everything was fine, including a blood sample I had given. Meanwhile I began to put items in the nursery. I sorted out books from our study which I had collected over many years and started to lovingly fold and store the baby items which had begun to come our way. Jenny, a colleague, re-covered a cushion and bouncing chair in the fabric I had chosen for the nursery; Nick's mother gave me presents every time I saw her; other friends and colleagues kindly gave me a huge range of gifts. I also began to buy toiletries and tiny clothes. I remember feeling very emotional when I bought the first packet of newborn nappies and even hugged the packet! I blossomed and was even pleased one day when someone said I looked fat!

The pregnancy became more real as each day passed. I received my official maternity leave letter from my employers and arranged for Nick and me to attend some 'National Childbirth Trust' (NCT) classes. We were disappointed to learn that Nick was only to be given three days' paternity leave so just hoped the baby would be 'on time' and arrive on the specific Friday it was due so he could have the weekend as a bonus. In early February I began a kick chart and found myself counting many times. Unusually we had a heavy snowfall and hardly any children came into school one day, so I made the most of the time chasing up my paperwork and making sure that everything was in place before my maternity leave was due to start on 16 March. My assistants kept reminding me to slow down because I would not even stop for breaks. I insisted I was fine. A couple of days later I was very tearful and did not know why. I went for my 28-week check-up feeling unwell and was sent to hospital by the midwife for tests as she had detected a urinary tract infection (UTI) in my water sample. She kindly explained that it was probably the cause of my tearful state at the time, the first since becoming pregnant. I did not like coming down from my permanent high. I was told the full test results would take a few days and in the meantime I should rest. The next day there was great excitement as we collected the pram we had ordered from the shop. It was a present from my parents. It was a lovely blue and white 'three-in-one' version. I spent ages working out how all the pieces came on and off, the different positions and imagining our baby in it. Even Nick practised pushing it.

My excitement was short-lived as next morning I felt very poorly. The doctor came out to see me and advised rest. However, I ended up rolling around half the night, absolutely screaming in agony with back and abdominal pains. Nick and I were very worried and scared. I was rushed off to hospital in the early hours of the morning by ambulance. The drive to our chosen maternity unit, about 20 minutes away, seemed like hours, and with the excruciating pains in my back I was sure I was about to lose the baby. The paramedics were very kind and offered me oxygen. I was panicking and just wanted Nick who was following behind in the car. Once at the hospital I felt more relaxed and relieved that I would be in safe hands. A nurse came to see me and I was connected to the heart-beat monitor (a sound which was to be heard regularly from then on). At least the baby was alive, I remember thinking. Nick and I were then left for what seemed like ages, with me still spasmodically rolling around in agony and my husband looking terrified. Eventually the door opened and a male doctor and nurse, who we had never seen before, appeared. I was briefly asked where the pain was and the next second the doctor snapped on a rubber glove, threw back the bed cover, lifted up my night dress and gave me an internal examination with no warning or explanation – all in front of my startled husband! We managed to explain that blood tests from the previous days had indicated a kidney infection. I felt shocked and upset by such abrupt treatment and very little was said before we were left alone again to worry further, although I was given some strong pain relief.

After several hours I was admitted to the antenatal ward where I stayed for ten days. One moment I would be chatting to another patient then the lower back pains would build and build. Often it took another patient to alert a nurse who would come and check on me. It then seemed ages before a doctor came, a different one each time, and through my pain I had to tell my story all over again. It made me feel like a fraud. After the worry and weakness of more pain I would be 'written up' for more morphine, then survive until the next attack. I had an intravenous line inserted in my hand and was surprised at how uncomfortable it was. The stiff piece of plastic that holds the needle in place is like a huge splinter and having a drip attached makes getting comfortable impossible. Every other patient in my bay of six beds had a consultant at their bedside at some point and I could hear their advice and programme of treatment as appropriate. My named consultant never appeared and I lurched from one attack to another. At one point they thought I may have kidney stones but this was not the case. One good thing was that I had another scan and was pleased to see a good profile of 'Baby H' who looked cute.

During my stay I experienced a whole range of nursing techniques, from midwives and nurses, and grew fond of those who had a smile and sympathy and not keen on those who scowled and had little patience with any of us in the room. I saw other pregnant women with a whole range of problems, usually high blood pressure, and others in initial stages of labour. I saw the cool, calm and collected ladies who walked around their beds breathing controlled, slow breaths. Then I saw and heard those who moaned, screamed and complained that they did not want an internal examination! I knew which way I wanted to be when my time came. The day after we would see 'Mum' and newborn walking in the corridor and a stream of happy people visiting them laden with bobbing 'new baby' helium balloons and gifts. It all looked so easy and problem free, just like the magazines and books implied. I felt that this stay in hospital had given me a great deal of insight into the whole procedure of 'birth' and began to read my magazines with a greater knowledge and confidence. As the days went by in hospital I slowly began to feel better and was discharged on 21 February.

I treated myself to a massage at home with a professional masseur and felt very relaxed and rejuvenated. Unfortunately I was weak from my stay in hospital so could not go back to work. The presents continued to flow in, lifting my spirits with each parcel. I had another scan which showed an even clearer profile of the baby who appeared to be sucking its thumb, a regular sight even to this day. I had knitted a bonnet and helmet in the smallest size. I did not want to know the sex of the baby beforehand but wanted the lovely surprise as it was born. I really wanted a girl as I have always been close to my mother and wanted a similar relationship with a daughter of my own. I wanted to buy pretty dresses and play at christenings in her bedroom. However, equally I wanted a boy as I hoped to have a second child and that could be a girl. I had loved having an older brother so my daughter would too! I also imagined a 'baby Nick' and thought how lucky I would be having two!

I saw the midwife at our local surgery who was a bit concerned as one of my routine tests showed problems again. Two days later I was back to hospital, again by ambulance. It took an hour to arrive as the paramedics had been given the wrong address. The same procedures occurred, i.e. still no consultant, left alone for long periods of time, lack of information about my problems. At least for this visit I knew all the 'kit' I needed, such as a mini Swiss army knife for trimming flowers and a whole range of tasks; a tiny salt cellar to liven up the food; a small jar of coffee (they only served tea); my own bottled water and unbreakable glass (I never felt that the jugs of water which were provided looked clean) and change for the phone. It seemed I had a urine infection and had to wait for the antibiotics to work. I made friends this time with another pregnant lady, called Jeannie, who was also in and out of hospital. We compared our stories and spent many hours chatting together and getting to know each other. Once discharged I felt much better this time and soon arranged to have my hair cut, filling in my hairdresser with some of the details of the past weeks. I had been going to the same salon for several years and Richard, my stylist, had begun to know me well, although no doubt he preferred the parachute jumping days than the current pregnancy tales. I wonder why women tell their hairdressers their life-story?

As part of my desire to research and learn as much as possible about childbirth, Nick and I had been to one of the NCT classes at one of their member's homes. This is a group who believe in natural birth techniques and teach you some of the methods to cope with them, e.g. massage and breathing deeply. After the child is born they offer excellent advice and support for breast-feeding and general postnatal help. Nick and I wanted him to be present at the birth and therefore he was keen to learn about his potential role too. Unfortunately, we were not impressed though as some of the other fathers treated it like a fun session in the pub, probably because they felt embarrassed. Possibly our values and ideas about the birth also differed from theirs. We believed that it should be private, dignified and with a relaxed but efficient approach. Others at this course appeared not to feel this way and obviously had the right and choice not to, but there seemed little point in sharing our ideas with them. We missed a few more sessions due to my hospital stays but decided they were not for us anyway.

I continued preparing the nursery even more by freshly washing everything and packed my hospital case according to all the literature I had read, down to the Evian facial spray and bed socks! We bought a cot bed, assembled it in the nursery and I placed baby items in it. One day my son or daughter would be in it – at last my dream was to be fulfilled.

At my next appointment as an outpatient at the local hospital, I actually saw a consultant who was a very efficient lady I had overheard seeing patients whilst on the wards. She was appalled when I told her my history and could not understand why no one had told her about me whilst I was in as she specialised in kidney problems in pregnancy. I had another scan that showed the baby was fine and weighed about four pounds.

In mid-March I finished work officially and went into school for the afternoon. I received a teddy bear which played lullabies and flowers from the staff. Unfortunately I was also back on more antibiotics for another urinary infection! My nesting instinct continued and I had decided I would do my bit for the environment and use non-disposable nappies which duly arrived by post. I also found some tiny coat hangers and took great delight in hanging up all the baby clothes. The co-ordinated (of course) pram bag was ordered too. I now looked and felt very pregnant and, being on true maternity leave now, wanted to make the most of it. I joined an aqua-natal class at a leisure centre and loved being with other expectant mums and comparing experiences. For a first-time mother, I felt like I had 'insider' knowledge due to my two stays on the antenatal ward. I also attended a parent-craft class at my health centre. These ran over a six-week period which you began in the final couple of months of pregnancy. I was so keen I arrived a week too soon and joined the reunion gathering of a previous group! One new mother of four weeks was already wearing her size ten white jeans again, much to the envy of everyone else. They recalled their birth stories, all of which sounded just like the books, and further confirmed that I knew what to expect. How I longed to be holding my baby, especially when my friend Jeannie, whom I had met in hospital, rang to say she had given birth to a son.

Meanwhile, I carried on being quite busy, although my moods had begun to swing from me being happy and excited one minute, then tearful the next. I saw my consultant who said it was a small baby but that she had no concerns, much to my relief. To celebrate this relatively good news Nick and I went to one of our 'courting' restaurants for a meal with a colleague who was leaving work. I felt very romantic sitting there as I was so pleased to be happily married and pregnant. The following morning I was up at 5.30 a.m., ironing, as I could not sleep! I then had a very energetic day in spite of the early start by going to my old class group for a special meal at school, then on to a parent-craft class at the health centre.

When the midwives were telling us about the hospital routines I was able to add comments from my experience and warned the other ladies to take the extra items I had needed. My knowledge was useful when I went on the official hospital tour to show me the delivery rooms and water birth suite. I loved the suite and decided I wanted a water birth. The whole maternity unit was due for upgrading and the only completed area was this one, with new decor and furnishings. The only other lady on the tour seemed to know nothing about the birth, equipment or anything. I felt like an expert because I had read the books and been on the antenatal ward! Afterwards I called to see my friends, Janet and Kevin, from college. They had a little boy who was almost one and they loaned me his wicker Moses basket and baby carrier. The Moses basket was a full-sized version of a tiny one I had had as a child. Yet again I felt my dream was coming true.

Soon it was April, the month that our baby was due. One day Nick and I were visited by his friends and we went out for a meal. I felt blooming and secretly hoped that we may bump into my ex-husband who lived locally to the pub, but we did not. The last few weeks I kept myself busy with shopping for baby items, including a stand for the Moses basket and a net as we had two cats and I was worried they may get into the basket. I bought and soon used more wool for baby clothes. I went to my friend Jeannie's, whom I had met in hospital, for lunch and enviously cuddled Oliver, her tiny newborn son. One day I called at my parent's house where I got the urge to clean their conservatory from top to bottom! My mother had finished a shawl which she had been doing since September. It was a beautiful masterpiece, so delicate in three-ply wool. I ached to hold my baby in it.

After three days of nagging stomach pains I phoned the hospital and once again I was admitted. I had a very long night and hardly slept. To occupy myself I knitted another tiny cardigan. As I worked on a sleeve all I could hear was another patient in labour. I was so jealous and wished so much it could be me. I do not think I have ever knitted with such vengeance before or since! Twenty-four hours later I was back at home and slept like a log – a big one. At the next antenatal class we had a talk from the health visitors about their role. Little did I know then how much I would be seeing of them.

I filled the next week by adding to my nursery stocks even more. I bought a breast pump, which was another vital piece of equipment according to my books and I knew I wanted to breast-feed my baby. I went for groceries, to a craft fair and to Marks and Spencer. The only relaxation I had was to choose some photograph albums for our wedding pictures. It was a job I had never got round to and filling them was a very therapeutic and enjoyable task. My nights were becoming increasingly sleepless either through pains, heartburn or merely being so big and uncomfortable. One morning I admit to being very rude to religious callers who woke me to ask me how I felt about the state of the world when it seemed I had only just managed to get to sleep! I spent the rest of the day cleaning our cooker, a task I had intended doing since we had moved in. I was pleased I had this urge as it fitted with the 'nesting' instinct described by my books as being part of the final stages of pregnancy, so I must be near its end.

Then it was time for another trip to the hairdresser. I remember making this appointment and hoping I would not make it. I did, but it was still a treat as Richard and his staff always made me feel good. My hair was in great condition too and the longest it had been for years. I had lunch out with my parents then we went to collect my pram bag. I was getting very impatient now for this baby! The Saturday before I had the baby Nick and I were busy shopping for a telephone, a nursing bra and more toiletries. We then trailed to one side of the county for a new holly tree then to the other side to collect the hanging baskets we had ordered. Not surprisingly I then had another bad night and felt tired and sore all the next day. On the Monday my mother and I went to Altrincham and bought a pram parasol and more pram sheets. I now had sore feet which were beginning to swell. It was probably due to all this shopping! I spent Tuesday with my friend Sue and her baby Ben, then on to a 'Mums and Tots' group at her church. I had first met Sue through 'Rotaract' and then we had worked together when I moved to the local special school. From then on we had become firm friends, especially as we were having children around the same time. After tea Nick and I walked up to the local hill and church grounds for some fresh air. It is only about 60 metres from our house, up a steep cliff. From the top you can see across Runcorn to Widnes and Liverpool and over to Chester and Wales. On a clear day you can spend hours 'just looking' and we find it peaceful and fascinating. Despite the fresh air and being busy it was another bad night for lack of sleep.

I had a lie-in, unusually, but managed to get to the parent-craft class about jabs and safety. One of the midwives also briefly mentioned postnatal depression and the possible symptoms. She reassured us that it was rare and would be checked up on by the health visitors. In our group of ten ladies there was only one who was not expecting for the first time. Her first son was now about six and she decided she wanted to be reminded about the parent-craft skills. She had quite a pessimistic approach to most subjects and I think the rest of us had almost begun to expect negative comments from her about everything. I remember her comment that she had had postnatal depression after her first child and I know I was not alone in thinking 'Typical, she's just the type!' How I would live to regret and learn from that thought.

The next day several people phoned to ask how I was and to ask if there was any sign of the baby. I felt irritable and even more impatient. My mother suggested we had lunch in town along with my grandmother. I went but did not feel hungry. Then we went into IKEA, a furniture store. I felt very weary and tired. At one point they found me just sitting on a pile of rugs! My grandmother tells me that this is an image she always has of me as she knew then her great grandchild's arrival was imminent. After tea I went to a DIY store with Nick. Did I never give up? At bedtime I thought I had a 'show' due to a pink stain. After a few restless hours I eventually woke Nick at 4.30 a.m. The pains were becoming stronger – was this it?

During the last few difficult and painful weeks many people, including medical staff, friends and relatives, had said to me, 'Oh, because you've been through all this the birth will be a doddle.'

They had convinced me. My mother had not had any problems, so why should I? All the time I was still so excited and I could not wait to feel the baby in my arms. Over the next few hours I felt like all I had ever dreamed of was about to come true and the first real labour pains were of joy, not suffering.

CHAPTER 3

The birth

The main part of the birth I really looked forward to was the moment they lay the baby on you. I imagined it being similar to the exhilaration of feeling the bare body next to you of your newly-wed husband. I expected pain, but I realised one or two other women had been through childbirth so I guessed I would be okay too! My mother had said that at least you know that the pain will end; you know what is causing it and you are rewarded by a beautiful child. I did not mind which gender, just as long as the child was healthy. Being teachers of disabled children possibly makes it worse, knowing the tremendous impact such a child can have on a family. Equally we did not know what a 'normal' child was, except I knew I wanted one. So when I actually went into labour I was so excited because I knew it was finally happening.

I started contractions about one or two in the morning on my expected delivery date. I practised the walking around and breathing that I had observed during the nights in hospital, feeling so pleased that at last I was to be a mum. Around 4.30 a.m. I decided to wake Nick. He had begun to sleep in the spare room since my hospital stays as I was restless at night and needed to spread out with my bump. We phoned the hospital ward and they suggested I had a bath and if I was still having pains to come in for 7 o'clock.

On the drive to the hospital we joked about being in labour on the expected date as Nick is renowned for his punctuality and 'being in good time'. All along he had said I would have this baby on a Friday teatime, because it fitted in time wise. It was a suitable day to miss school and then to have the weekend, leaving his precious paternity-leave days for the homecoming.

Once we arrived at the hospital Nick found me a wheelchair and left me to 'check in' whilst he parked the car. I was having contractions but they were not too painful, numbed by my excitement I think. We were put into a side room and waited for the usual checks which we were both now quite accustomed to – the bleep of the heart monitor and internal inspections by a sensitive midwife. Eventually by 9 o'clock she declared I was sufficiently dilated to go into the water birth suite which was available. They had the staffing to cover it and there seemed to be no problems with the baby or me. These reasons had been given to me previously for not being able to use it and I was even more pleased to have got this far.

I opted for a water birth as I had seen the suite for it and thought 'Oh, yes please'. It was by far the best room in the labour ward so I had to have it! In the magazines the water births looked so easy, almost transcendental with a 'closest to nature' appeal, complete with incense burning, wind-chimes and a relaxed-looking husband! I walked down the corridor to the suite and put a few things in the en-suite bathroom and 'made home', one of my favourite aspects of going away. All my kit was there and every possible item recommended to make it all so wonderful and easy. Nick took a couple of photographs of me by the 'pool' which reminded me of a jacuzzi in a posh hotel. I did not want any more photographic evidence from this point. The midwife filled the pool with warm water and when it was full and at the right temperature I took off my nightdress and got in. The pains were like teenage years period pains – waiting to be soothed by a hot water bottle and a sympathetic mother.

The first part of the birth was just as I had imagined. The warm water was definitely soothing and I was very happy that it was all about to happen. I had asked Nick to let our families and colleagues know that I had gone in and I remember thinking that they would be excited too. The midwife was lovely and chatted to us both about many topics. As the labour pains became stronger she gave me gas and air to breathe. She had put the radio on in the room and I remember moving to the rhythm of the beat of a song by George Michael, concentrating on breathing and getting high, declaring, 'Oh, I can see now why they say giving birth is like sex – this is purely orgasmic!'

Meanwhile Nick and the lovely, pretty midwife were chatting about different topics, including the need to be well stocked at home with spare toilet rolls! In my euphoric state I remember thinking that it would be nice for our baby to be greeted by such a sweet face and endearing smile. It seemed strange moving around this small pool, totally naked and having 'messy bits' fished out with a net by an attractive lady talking to your husband – almost surreal but not unpleasant. I was just glad she was so chatty and she and Nick had a relaxed (as far as possible) chat. I was getting higher on the gas and air but more uncomfortable as the pains became stronger and more regular, but I was still happy and aware of everything which was going on. Nick kept passing me drinks and mopping my brow (just like the magazines) and at one stage my consultant visited us. She had never seen the pool in use before. She wished us well and said she would see us again soon. So far so good. However, as I became fully dilated and my waters broke, the midwife saw there was meconium (baby excrement) in the water, an indication that the baby was not happy, so I had to get out. That is where my ideal version of birth ended.

The baby was stuck and in distress. I had become so exhausted because I had been awake all night, then in the pool for four hours. After being in hot water all that time I was very, very weary, and when it came to actually pushing, my body could not do it. The midwife had called for more staff to help. The intimate calmness of the pool, chat and music was replaced by feeling very cold on a delivery bed with what seemed like a sea of panicking faces around me and shouting at me to 'push'. My exhausted body just could not get the hang of pushing at all, and everyone still seemed to be shouting at me – who were all these strangers? I remember saying to Nick, 'I've had enough – take me home now. That's it, let's go.'

I then moved on to shouting 'Get this thing out of me!' That inspired me a little as I remembered at the antenatal classes they said once you got to the abusive stage you were almost there. Yet I just could not seem to co-ordinate the muscles required for pushing the baby out. I know they let me feel the baby's head, but with each four pushes I only had one effective one. I heard someone say that if I did not do it soon then I would have to have an emergency Caesarean. Another voice tried to describe to me again which muscles I should push with and I tried to visualise the pictures and models I had been shown of a birth. I was half sitting up and seemed to have staff either side of me and some others between my legs, all telling me what I should do. There seemed to be a frightening sense of urgency that I was powerless to control. I think Nick was by me most of the time, holding my hand, and in the occasional moment I was mentally functioning I know he looked really scared. It felt like being really drunk for the first time when you are spinning from the enjoyment level to the illness and regret stage. In between, the pain level was far beyond anything I had ever experienced before and apparently it was too late to give me any pain relief. I began to dread the wave of pain as it built then crashed into my abdomen with an enormous jolt.

They decided at last that an episiotomy was needed and a local anaes-thetic was given. As they waited for it to take effect and let go of me for a few seconds (probably to let their hands recover from me squeezing them), I felt the tremendous urge to push. I widely gesticulated with my arms for support and managed to combine all my efforts into getting everything co-ordinated. I was vaguely aware of the chubby arm and feel of a midwife on my right side, a complete stranger who shared the most intimate moment of my life. I do not even know what she looked like but I appreciated all she did. Then eventually they gave me a slight cut and at the final stage I did get it right and the baby was born, to everyone's relief. Our original midwife delivered him, declared we had a little boy and I waited to feel his little body on mine, but immediately they whisked him off to the other side of the room. My immediate feelings were mixed: slight disappointment it was not a girl; relief I had eventually delivered him but then immense anti-climax of not feeling him next to me. It was as if I had just made passionate love and I had been left lying there naked, without a kiss, as my lover abruptly left the room.

Nick kissed me and we were told that the baby was a very funny colour.

Apparently the cord had been round his neck and he was not breathing. So straight away I did not get that initial bond that I had been looking forward to. I still feel a real pang of regret at that and for a long time I could not bear to watch birth scenes on television. The baby was treated by two paediatricians who cleared his airway and I heard the first, of many, cries. He was wrapped up and taken out of the room as apparently they wanted to check his colour in daylight. As the other staff seemed to vanish we commented that he had been born at 3.09 p.m., just as we had hoped. I immediately felt 'sober' and told Nick to phone our mothers and school. He said there was no rush but he was told otherwise by me! I cannot remember even holding our baby son by this stage as he was still out of the room. I think both Nick and the baby were back in the room as I began to drift back into semi-consciousness.

I had apparently a postpartum haemorrhage. Nick said blood just gushed out, soaking through the bed and creating pools on the floor. I had a retained placenta. It was like a scene from the television drama *Casualty*. They had buzzed for another paediatrician to attend to the baby who they were still concerned about; they were also buzzing in more staff for me. I felt the staff were beginning to panic as one then another tried to make me push out the placenta, but my body could take no more. I remember thinking that I did not realise about having to push out the placenta. I thought it just naturally came out. Then they said I needed emergency surgery and I vaguely heard voices trying to phone for a theatre and more doctors. I felt I was being pulled and prodded from every direction yet I became detached from it. I seemed to float around the room above everyone and felt I was watching the scene from above.

Nick said there was just blood everywhere. I remember feeling very, very cold. Icy cold. I began to shiver violently. Words like 'theatre', 'emergency' and 'right now' floated around the room along with a vague concept that all this had something to do with a baby. What baby? Whose baby? I did not have one. He had gone. More faces. More panic. More floating and drifting in and out of consciousness. Doors banging. Shouting out, 'I'm cold, so cold.' They threw Nick's big towelling dressing gown on me (packed in case he had joined me in the pool). Doors opened, bodies around me. Being wheeled. Someone said, 'Your son is waving.' I had a brief moment of full consciousness just enough to raise my eyes to see my darling Nick standing there holding our baby in his arms and getting him to wave. The look of horror and pain in my husband's eyes at that split second will never be erased from my memory.

Lights on the ceiling. More doors banging. More faces over me in masks. Tap on the hand and I was gone, sinking into blackness . . .

After I was wheeled off Nick and the baby seemed to have been forgotten about, I found out later. No one came to him in the suite and he just wandered around aimlessly, not knowing how I was or what to do with the baby. He placed him in a cot, tidied up our belongings, took a few photographs and just waited. Eventually a cleaner came in and looked very surprised to see them both there. Nick chatted to her as she cleaned out the tub and mopped up the pools of blood on the floor. At last a midwife came to weigh the baby, clean and dress him and place him back in the plastic cot. She took them through to an empty side room and he waited again.

I eventually came round, hours later, with drips everywhere. I had a catheter. I had blood transfusions. I just remember wires everywhere and bleeping machines. As I came to and opened my eyes, I was aware I was in a dimly lit room and felt like I had fallen from a great height. My whole body felt sore. It suddenly dawned on me that I had had the baby! I looked around to see poor Nick who was at my side looking ashen.

A different midwife came in, introduced herself, and checked my monitors and that I was comfortable. She then gently placed our baby in my weary arms and left us alone. At last I was holding *my* baby! He was apparently fine and I would be too. The cheery, kind midwife returned and took our first family photograph and Nick took some too of me and the baby. I could not move and had a dry mouth so on the nurse's suggestion Nick went to the hospital shop and bought me an iced lollipop. He then fed me with it from a spoon as I lay down and held drinks for me whilst I sipped from a straw. I was not sure of what had happened to me during the birth. I felt upset that there had been problems but I was just glad to be awake and calm after all the drama of the birth.

My thoughts turned to my parents whom I knew would be waiting excitedly to see their grandson and me, but I decided I did not want them to see me in the state I was in with all these wires. Luckily the nurse said, 'Oh no, no visitors today at all.' I wanted their first sight to be a pleasure, not the shock of me looking like a battle victim with hair like Medusa!

Our son was a pretty little thing. I know everyone thinks that of their newborn, but he really was. He weighed just under seven pounds and had delicate features, not a chubby creature at all. When Nick left, the midwife returned frequently to check on my every need and kept the baby right by me. I could not move due to all the wires so she gently propped me up on a few pillows. With my knees raised up a little I lay with him facing me. I spent hours just watching him sleep and examining every bit of him. He was *my* baby! It was a magical moment for me and I tried to capture it on film. On the actual photograph he looks all out of proportion though due to the angle of the camera. I just held him most of the night as I could not sleep properly. The midwife had shown the baby and I the correct position for breast-feeding. Our first few attempts were awkward although the baby instinctively suckled, but I felt strangely numb to the sensations. I was enjoying my initial hours of being a mother but it did not seem real somehow. In retrospect I guess I was just in shock.

The birth had been horrific for both Nick and I. We were robbed too of that precious moment after birth when the mother holds the child with father looking on for the first time and saying something romantic. Was I being too optimistic or am I right that it does happen like that for some people? I was still apparently on the delivery ward so must still be a concern to the staff. I knew from previous stays in the maternity unit that you went up to the ward very soon after the birth if all was well, so I must be a problem! It was apparently a quiet night as regards other deliveries. I could only hear faint voices and the occasional shout in the distance. I was glad I did not have to listen to the sounds of another birth.

Meanwhile I was still bleeding and discharging heavily. It is the nearest I have felt to being incontinent as an adult. It was reassuring though to have the same midwife to keep cleaning me up. She was so gentle, sensitive and kind, dealing with my unpleasant condition discreetly and efficiently. I appreciated her skill and manner very much. Eventually I was brought some breakfast, my first meal since Thursday evening. I ate it after being encouraged that I needed to eat for the baby. I had managed feeding him a few times too, but did not particularly feel excited by the sensation. The baby did appear to suckle well. I had expected my breasts to feel hard and full, but they just felt soft. My stomach still looked and felt huge though!

A doctor came to see me (a different one) and told me how lucky I had been yesterday. Lucky? I would not have called it that! He said if it had been a home birth or even 30 years ago in hospital I probably would not have survived. That shocked me and a lump came into my throat as I thought of how Nick had looked as they wheeled me off to theatre. Imagine if I had never woken up. I decided not to think that way. He checked me over and said I could have all the tubes removed as everything seemed fine. Once I had showered he told the nurse I could go up to the ward. Hurray!

Very slowly and carefully she helped me sit up, then stand. I realised then I had white, elasticated stockings on – very sexy! These were apparently to prevent blood clots. In the shower room she helped me undress and left me to wash. Little by little my body came back to life. I felt weary, ached and generally sore but only had one small wound to heal from the episiotomy. All my beauty kit, so carefully packed, was now put to use, but it is amazing just how much washing your hair and showering can drain you after such an event.

The nurses helped me back to my room and even rubbed moisturiser on my back – bliss! I could not cope with drying my thick hair properly so just tied it back. With every minute I felt my spirits rise and by the time we were wheeled up to the ward I was ecstatic. I was in the maternity ward with my beautiful baby! I was a mum! The birth had been horrible but I was trying my best to overcome it and as quickly as I could. So less than 24 hours later, there I was looking immaculate, wearing a bit of make-up and awaiting visitors.

CHAPTER 4

First days on the ward

We joined five other new mothers and babies in a bay in one of the two postnatal wards. I was a bit disappointed not to be on the other maternity ward at the opposite end of the corridor where I had been for antenatal stays. There seemed to be a friendly competitive element between the two wards and I admit I had liked the other ward and wanted to share these few special days with the staff who had nursed me before. In retrospect maybe I could have asked to be moved but at the time it did not seem too important. I did not really establish any close links with any of the people on the ward this time. Perhaps we were all too busy with our newborns instead of killing time with magazines and chatting.

I 'made home' once again sorting out my locker, fed and changed the baby again, had some lunch and eagerly awaited visitors. Was this the same person who had been attached to wires and monitors 12 hours earlier? To my parents and sister who soon arrived they must have thought Nick had been lying when he discouraged them from visiting the night before as 'it wasn't convenient' (I don't think they have ever forgiven him!). Yet this was just how I wanted them to meet the new baby. There I was looking immaculate, proud and thrilled to show him off. Naturally they were delighted and he was passed around. The first stream of beautiful cards and gifts arrived. My father put his specs on his new grandson and declared that he looked like Granny Hanzak!

Nick obviously came back too and was amazed to see the transformation in me from the night before. More flowers, cards and gifts. We sorted out the birth announcement cards, already addressed pre-hospital. One aspect was missing – the baby's name. For weeks previously we had both made a list of our favourite names for boys and girls and got down to a short list of six. Before Nick left that night I think I decided he was to be 'Dominic Marius', my choice, as I had suffered the pain! His first name was chosen because as a young teenager I had loved a Sunday afternoon BBC historical drama about smugglers in Cornwall – the hero was played by an actor called Dominic, a handsome young man with curly hair and who often wore a wonderful white, romantic shirt! My favourite musical is *Les Miserables* and its hero is called Marius. So now I had my own little hero.

Left alone after the day-long visiting I began to realise that all the other babies seemed to have long periods of sleep, allowing their mothers to rest.

Not mine! My baby seemed to cry all the time. He constantly wanted feeding and constantly wanted fussing. At one point the midwife said to me, 'He's like a little bird this one, forever wanting food.'

The first night on the ward I kept him with me in his crib, a plastic box really which looked like a fish tank. If you moved your baby anywhere you had to wheel them in it for safety reasons. He did not settle in it. They even put him in the bed next to me but just as I kept dropping off, he would wake up. By about 4 a.m. the night staff suggested they took him into the nursery for a while so I could get some sleep. Just as I drifted off the others' babies then started! Another night with little sleep.

Of course on Sunday morning Dominic slept beautifully back in the ward, but there was far too much noise from everything else for me to rest at all. We had more visitors initially – Nick's mother (now christened Granny H), Glenys (Nick's sister) and her son Patrick. More gifts and photographs. My mother-in-law had warned me that she would not want to hold the new baby as she felt insecure with his size. It did not mean she did not care but preferred to wait until he was a little bigger. She did hold his hand a lot and I was not worried by her honesty. Later on came my grandparents. They were thrilled too and the new addition was a welcome relief from the worry we were all having about my grand-mother who had a cancerous growth on her scalp. Once again both Dominic and I were fine whilst we had visitors who were all keen to assist in any way. He then slept from visiting until 11.30 p.m. then kept me awake all night again in both the ward and nursery. The night staff were lovely and made me very welcome to sit with them whilst they fed other babies and chatted away. I had almost become accustomed to the small hours and felt relaxed in the dim lights and relative quietness. That pattern lasted for three or four nights as they did not want me to go home immediately. Then I found every time I could rest because Dominic was sleeping there would be something else to disturb me, like the cleaner every morning at six o'clock, 'bash!' with the bin. When I settled again there would be another disturbance. Then if my baby was not crying, another one was.

In the few peaceful periods Dominic did allow me I began his 'First Year: week by week diary'. This was a present from Claire. It was a lovely book with appropriate information on one side and space to write about your baby on the other. Just my cup of tea! On the first page I added my note at the bottom: 'Hospital musts: salt, coffee, water, money, disposable pants, Swiss army knife!'

I also noted in the diary that Dominic loved to be handled all the time, and feeding was going well initially. I began to learn about my son. I loved feeling his little body and watching him move. He had blue eyes and hair the same colour as mine. He had delicate, perfect features; the only blemish was a red 'V' on his forehead, apparently some babies get them from the pressure on their skull at birth. He fed impatiently at first, finding my nipple and then gulping fast. He seemed most wakeful mid-morning, mid-afternoon, early evening and in the night! His favourite sleeping position was on his back with his arms up by his ears. When awake he often put his fingers near his mouth. I wondered if he would become a thumb-sucker.

On the Monday morning the pretty midwife who had delivered him came up to see us both and teased me that her husband had complained when she was late home on Friday. One of the water suite conversations had been about how she often worked over her shift due to delayed arrivals and we had kept her for hours. It was lovely to see her and I managed to take a photograph of her with Dominic.

I gave my baby his first bath on the Monday morning in a green washing-up bowl! He gave me his first 'windy' smiles and had lots of clothes changes. I adored actually using the tiny clothes I had lovingly gathered for months. At one change I made the mistake of not keeping him covered as I changed his nappy and he urinated all over my bed. The nurse on duty was very offhand with me when I explained I needed it changing. My parents and Claire came again laden with gorgeous presents and flowers. Jeannie, my hospital friend, visited us too and brought a charming pale blue suit. She looked great and we congratulated ourselves on being proud mothers. Then I had another very sleepless night.

By the following morning I was getting very, very weepy because I was just so exhausted. I also had huge, hard lumps which felt like footballs in my armpits. They were sore and very uncomfortable. I thought at first I had an allergic reaction to my travel-size deodorant or something. Eventually when I told a nurse she told me that it was 'my milk coming in' and that it would not last long. I wished that the nurses would not underestimate my ignorance as a first-time mother! I might have read all the books but there was still a great deal I had to learn! It would have been better to have been told a fact five times than not at all as a great deal of concern and worry could have been avoided. Sometimes I felt that the nursing staff were too blasé about many typical aspects of newborn care and as new mothers you can feel inadequate and stupid. Often those who were very young seemed to cope better than some of us older and more educated women. There must be a lesson in that!

As the day progressed I felt very hot and my breasts felt on fire and dreadfully tender. I had developed mastitis, inflammation of the mammary gland. The prospect of another disturbed night on the ward was too much to bear and I pleaded with the sister, sobbing, 'Please can I have my own room as I just can't go on like this. I'm going to go home exhausted.'

I was given various reasons for this not being possible, such as the individual rooms being reserved for those with Caesarean deliveries and that they were all full. They just felt like mean excuses to me at that time! I suggested I went home but they said in view of the condition that I was in they did not recommend it. Luckily they did find me a room, and I had a 'do not disturb' note on the door.

Not long after we had moved my college friend, Janet, called with a lovely cotton 'Winnie the Pooh' outfit. It was wonderful to have privacy and quiet to ourselves and I was able to 'make home' yet again. Even Dominic had longer sleeps and good feeds all day, although it was painful for me. Nick appeared in the daytime as he had not gone to school. He looked grey and exhausted. I had gone back into an excited mode whilst he just seemed to sit and stare as I busied myself unwrapping more cards and examining presents. My parents and Claire came again and videoed us in the room. They brought even more presents. It amazed me that a new baby accumulated so many things in just a few days.

By that evening, physically and mentally, I improved. It was tremendous to actually have peace to settle when Dominic did. At least when he woke that night and I had fed and changed him no other baby would disturb us. He did not settle though so I decided I would go and see my night staff chums in the nursery for a while. I carried Dominic in my arms and as I emerged from the end of the dimmed corridor a nurse appeared from the room next to mine. She let me walk past her and followed me without saying a word. As we approached the lights and voices of the nursery she suddenly snapped at me, 'What on earth are you doing carrying your baby around? You know it is against hospital policy and *you* should know better!'

I mumbled something about not wanting to disturb other patients as the cribs were noisy to wheel but she snapped back, 'That is irrelevant – and what did you want anyway?'

'Just company,' was my pathetic reply, but I was told I should be sleeping! If only! With that she carried Dominic back to our room and I spent the next few hours sobbing and cuddling my baby. I could not understand why she had not stopped me when she first saw me to reprimand me gently, not scold me like a naughty child. I wanted to go home.

I drifted off to sleep at last and Dominic slept most of the morning again which gave me chance to get myself bathed. We were both checked over and told we could go home. Dominic weighed just over seven pounds, was feeding well and presented no problems. Equally they said I would soon settle down with the mastitis and so I excitedly packed up. I proudly put a white velour all-in-one suit on Dominic, which I had bought with my mother months earlier, specifically for this occasion. He also had a fleecy white suit that Granny H had sent in and of course the tiny white helmet I had knitted. I prefer a new baby in white, not denim or bright colours. I am a traditionalist and proud of it! I had asked Nick to bring in my white maternity polo shirt and grey pinafore dress. I knew I would not fit into my ordinary clothes as I was still very swollen. I put my make-up on too and, in spite of the tiredness, waited for our departure with eager anticipation.

Nick arrived and the midwife who had first bathed Dominic carried him down in the lift and out to the car for us. This procedure was hospital policy. She put him in his car seat and we set off for home, baby and me in the back. We were now a family!

CHAPTER 5

Coming home

I felt so excited on the quiet, 20-minute drive home from hospital. It was 1 May, cloudy but warm, and the thought of all the summer months at home with my baby was wonderful. When we arrived at our house a neighbour appeared and took the first family photograph of us on the drive. Nick and I look tired but happy. Dominic was asleep after his first car journey. We even took pictures inside the house with him in his car seat on the lounge rug – typical new parents. The lounge was soon filled with all the beautiful cards and presents we had received. After my first breast-feed at home Dominic fell asleep. I laid him on one of the settees surrounded by pillows. Both of our cats, Thomas and Jacob, were very interested and I was very jumpy, expecting them to suffocate him! Later on we lay him in his cot in his nursery whilst we sorted out places for all his new clothes and equipment. I was ridiculously happy opening things like cotton wool from my treasured collection that had been waiting for months to be used. Although we had a few 'welcome home' phone calls, no visitors came.

Nick and I had agreed that when I did come home, initially we would probably be in different bedrooms as I was going to be demand-feeding Dominic. Nick does not function well if he is short of sleep and as he would be at work and I would not then it made sense for me to cope with Dominic in the night. So from that first night he went in the spare bedroom with a single bed (the 'blue room', so-called due to the décor), and baby and I were in our big bedroom. The wicker crib I had been loaned looked ideal and surrounded by all the plush white bedding, Dominic looked angelic. It was a long first night with Dominic wanting a feed, change and contact on a regular basis. I hardly got any sleep but I knew it would get better . . .

The following morning the midwife and general practitioner (GP) called to see us both and check us over, with no problems. I remember thinking how blasé I had become about taking down my pants and letting people look! My mother had always said that once you had a baby then you lost your inhibitions about such things. I now understood her. Dominic howled when the doctor was with us and I heard myself making excuses that he was not always like this, but that he did seem to be quite demanding. My parents and grandparents visited us briefly and I resumed the usual tasks of washing and making a meal. At night we gave Dominic his first bath at home, in the washbasin. It went reasonably well. Both of us tackled it in our usual organised way with all the required equipment laid out and began to establish a routine. We discovered that our new baby monitor did not work when we put him to sleep upstairs whilst we attempted to watch television downstairs. All the baby literature and adverts attempt, and in most cases succeed, to convince you that all these gadgets are vital and without them your baby could suffer. Consequently I could not relax for fear of him choking, dying of cot death syndrome or being suffocated by the cats!

At a week old Dominic had his first trip out – shopping of course – and he slept throughout. The midwife called to see us again and check on feeding (fine) and sleeping (no comment). He also had a sleep in the re-covered bouncy chair from a relative. The lap strap was under his chin! Nick had taken to drinking a glass or two of red wine most evenings and we have a lovely photograph of him with glass in one hand and Dominic in the other with a 'what have we done?' expression on his face. Even though I was up with him during the night Nick was still hearing every sound and so was also getting very tired.

The next day was special as it was my grandparents' diamond wedding anniversary. Owing to my due date of delivery and my grandmother's ill health we had decided just to have a small party at my parents' home. Claire had gone back up to her home in Glasgow and Kevin was in Zimbabwe so it was just us three with my parents and grandparents. We took many photographs of us all in different situations around the house and garden and had a tasty meal. I often look at them and feel how happy I was at that stage. My hair is shining, my eyes sparkling and I was flushed with general contentment. My family all have doting expressions for their new grandson. As a child I had always hoped that my grandmother would live to see me get married. Not only had she done so twice but now here she was holding my child too – smashing! On the dark drive back home I was fascinated watching Dominic's eyes responding to the flashes from streetlights and how alert he looked. It had been a good day.

Over the first weekend his cord fell off and we felt more confident changing and washing him. Nick was very willing to help in his care and although at times I would feel a bit frustrated that he did not do it identi-cally to me, I did realise I should be grateful and that there is more than one way to change a nappy! If it did not leak then what was the problem? My concern for the environment and desire for using non-disposable nappies rapidly faded when I realised how convenient the disposable ones were. In Dominic's diary there was advice about 'postnatal blues'. I had read it and wrote 'I'm fine' next to it.

During the next few weeks we began to build a few routines to fit our new lifestyle. I do not think either of us really appreciated before his birth just how much everything would change. Suddenly our whole lives revolved around his every need. We both like to be tidy and organised and I rarely heeded advice that 'when baby rests, Mum does too'. If he had a sleep I would then want to tidy up, put a load of washing on or sort out the post. Just as I would feel ready to sit down Dominic would begin his loud shouts for attention and needs. We had plenty of visitors and I loved to show my baby off to them all.

I found the first few weeks as a mother exciting. I loved all the paraphernalia to be gathered before outings and the rigmarole involved. We took him to a local park, for his first pram trip on May Bank Holiday Monday. I was as proud as a dog with two tails pushing him around. I just felt rather frumpy as all I could wear were leggings and t-shirts. Of course we had packed all the necessary kit in the co-ordinating pram bag! The following day Nick returned to school leaving me alone with Dominic for the first time. It was another big step and I missed having my husband around. Yet I knew the coming weeks would seem short-lived and very precious so I thought positively to make the most of it.

I managed well for the first couple of days. I took him shopping locally and was really pleased to meet people I knew, so I could beam! With a brand new baby I soon realised how other people are attracted to you both and cannot resist the usual questions of 'How old is he?', 'Is he good for you?' and the ultimate comment 'They don't stay like that for long'. You do not realise how true this actually is until a few months later. Already Dominic was beginning to grow out of the smallest sized suits.

We had various friends who visited us along with the midwife and our health visitor, a pleasant young lady. Everyone always seemed to enquire how I was doing and naturally I felt everything was hunky dory. After one particularly bad night though I did ask my father to come round just so I could have a shower without worrying and I did admit that I needed an hour or so to myself. On a couple of walks that week Dominic had cried loudly, leaving me perplexed as to the cause as I had fed, winded and changed him. Why did he not settle like all the books say?

At two weeks old he had his first big bath with father! I had read that it was a good bonding experience for each of them as the baby would feel more secure with the bodily contact and their father would feel useful. All that happened for us was that Dominic screamed blue murder and Nick got terribly stressed! Forever the optimist, I said that it was bound to get better if we all persevered. All that Nick seemed to see of his son since his return to work was a wide, crying mouth demanding something with very little to enthuse about.

The next morning it was sunny and we had decided Nick would go for our usual bedding plants for the front garden and some baskets whilst Dominic and I slept. For once we both had a lie-in after our typically disturbed night and when I did surface I looked out of the kitchen window to see Nick planting the last flower in the front border. He came in a little later to find me hysterically in tears and gasping huge sobs. He presumed that I must have received terrible news but instead I accused him of being terribly mean and selfish. I yelled at him that did he not realise that all I had become was a feeding machine, a fat one at that; who had no life of her own any more; who could not get a night's sleep; who did not have intelligent conversations anymore and all she had looked forward to for days was a bit of time and space for herself to dig in the garden and plant bedding plants and let someone else change nappies for once!

I do not think I had ever literally shouted at Nick before and I am not sure who was more shocked at the outburst, him or me. At least he did the best thing and just hugged me whilst I cried and meekly said that he thought he had been being useful. We had a quiet relaxing day and a slightly better bath time. We even tried Dominic with water in a bottle to give me a break. I felt tired all day after my 'do' but better for a good cry.

The next day was still sunny so we had a pleasant family walk in a local forest and had a big roast dinner at my parents. It was my mother's idea to help us out. The 'Dad and sprog' bath was a big success too. Whilst I was pregnant Nick had called the bump 'sprog' many times and still used it! Dominic only officially objected to this just before he was five years old when he said he would not answer us if we called him that. Within those first two weeks he had also grown out of 'newborn' nappies. My milk was obviously doing him good.

Meanwhile I was still taking in all the hints and advice from his diary. This week's suggestion was to start some savings schemes for the baby. We duly opened a post office account for his money and decided to use his child benefit allowance towards a PEP savings scheme so he would have a 'nest egg' in later life.

One morning I had a major shock. Although I had read warnings that newborn babies should not be seated in bouncy chairs, I had ignored them. He seemed to like it and I felt he was safe and comfortable in it. Nick had gone to work this particular day and just before I decided to go upstairs and get dressed, I thought I would tidy up the kitchen. To keep my eye on Dominic I placed him carefully on one of the kitchen surfaces, in his chair, and began to put things away. In a split second, Dominic kicked his legs slightly and the chair, with him in it, fell to the floor! I screamed and turned it over immediately. Dominic was screaming; I was hysterical. I could not see any marks on his head but put a cold compress on regardless. This made him cry even more. I telephoned my father who arrived within minutes. I trusted his expertise in first aid and after checking my baby over, he said he was fine. We worked out that the strap would have held him in and the chair frame would have hit the floor and not his head. I was a dithering wreck but Dominic was calm and content again. My father encouraged me to have a hot drink and to have it whilst

I soaked in the bath. Thank heaven for grandfathers. Let this be a warning to others too!

After my outburst at Nick, I seemed a bit calmer in general and carried on with visits to various places. We went to my old class for a meal; more shopping; first clinic trip to be weighed; first Mums and Tots group with Sue and her baby Ben, where we were the centre of attention as the newest members. However, I had started to have considerable pain if I tried to go to the toilet, as if something was tearing inside, and I got very tearful about it. The midwife came for her last visit and I told her. She examined me and said it was just the tightness caused by my stitches healing up and would pass. By the following morning I was in agony and had to get an emergency appointment with the doctor. I was examined and informed that I did have several tears around my anal passage and vagina which were a little infected and if I pushed to pass a motion then they were all ripping further. She was amazed the midwife had not detected it the day before but reassured me that if I applied the cream she prescribed along with a lactulose-based softening agent then it would all heal within a week or so.

At the weekend we visited Nick's family. Granny H still did not hold the baby but took plenty of photographs instead of her two grandsons, Patrick and Dominic. We then called to see my friends, Debbie and Alan, where Dominic was sick all over me and we had to make a hasty retreat home. Nick and I were both now increasingly tired by both day and night happenings. Each evening we tried to settle him down reasonably early in an attempt to have some time to ourselves, only to be woken at 1 a.m. and 4.30 a.m. for an hour each time. This was beginning to be almost a pattern. That Sunday my parents took him away from me for the first time to show him to their friends. The plan was for me to rest but I could not settle, so ended up doing silly chores instead, bemoaning that I did not like him away from me!

The following week consisted of more visitors, including our head teacher, and more shopping trips. At home I still persisted in doing housework whilst Dominic slept. He had begun to occasionally stop crying if he heard my voice, almost copied me if I smiled and had begun to bang at items dangling from his play gym. I also discovered that he would go to sleep if I danced to Michael Bolton with him. Was this because he recognised it from the concert we went to before he was born? One night he had us both awake from 2.30 a.m. to 5 a.m., and then poor Nick had to go into work.

When the health visitor came, I had various points lined up for her (answers in italics):

- Were we trying too hard or too early to get him into an evening routine? *No real answer.*

- I was getting engorged again. *She advised that I expressed some milk.* (Several painful attempts with a buzzing, battery-operated breast pump only succeeded in about 5 ml and plenty of frustrated tears!)
- Could we now try gripe water to see if that would calm his cries? *Yes.*
- Was the lump on Dominic's left nipple normal? *Yes, he still had some female hormones in him.*

I found it useful that someone would visit and you could ask them such questions.

My sister Claire came home from Scotland for the weekend and whilst Nick stayed in, cleaning out all the kitchen cupboards (his way of relaxing), we went into Warrington and experienced a selection of 'mother and baby' changing rooms – Boots having the best. My nipples felt very sore and my breasts like enormous watermelons. During the night my temperature shot up and Nick called out the GP next morning. She confirmed I had mastitis again with a bad infection. More medication and a few days in bed were called for.

By the end of his first month Dominic weighed 9 lb 10 oz and was 5 cm longer than at birth. He had a varied sleep pattern but tended to wake at midnight, 3 a.m. and 6 a.m. When he was hungry he had no patience, so I was glad to breast-feed him as it was always 'on tap' and at the correct temperature. His head control was improving, his skin was paler and he had lost some of his initial hair. I had begun to know his different cries for hunger, pain and generally being niggly. His response to me was 'feed me' but sometimes I could soothe him. His usual response to his father was to fill his nappy and/or squawk!

This was our first taste of family life and it was proving more demanding than all the books and magazines implied...

CHAPTER 6

Another hospital stay

During that Whitsuntide week I slowly recovered from mastitis, helped by Nick being at home for half-term. We were able to complete a few small tasks around the house, making us both feel a little more human again. Without the work routine for either of us our whole pace seemed easier. We even shared the same bedroom for a couple of nights. We all went to register Dominic's birth, which was a pleasurable trip as he looked immaculate and was content (for once). It was the same registrar who had married us which somehow seemed right. On various other trips out, fitted in around Dominic's needs, I ended up feeding him in a selection of different car parks. Why did he not do what all the books stated he should and, for example, now be into a settled sleeping routine? We did manage a social night out as a family when we went to Sue and her husband Jon's house for their joint 30th birthday party. I was pleased to show off our baby as he was as good as gold, sleeping on their bed from 9 p.m. to 1.30 a.m. when we went home. Shame he was awake then most of the night!

The following day we met up with my college friends, Margaret and Richard, who had a son, Oliver, almost exactly twelve months older than Dominic. Obviously I could not help but compare his progress to Dominic's. He had slept through from about two weeks of age, was no trouble at all and would lie contentedly for ages without demanding anything. The difference between them currently was vast too. I began to feel that we must be doing everything wrong. On the positive side we had noticed that Dominic had begun to look at items more and for longer periods, like the black and white cot book; he had started to touch objects like the 'Noddy' dangling from his pram and his gym toys. He would also grab at my hair and Nick's shirts. Yet he still would not settle to sleep for long and when he was awake he would want constant attention. I resisted leaving him crying for very long because I felt he was still very young and would surely improve soon.

Luckily Nick had a two-week Whitsuntide holiday from school that year and I was able to leave Dominic with him whilst I went to see the consultant for my postnatal check at our local hospital. The last time I had seen her was in my 'high' time in the water birth suite and she began by just congratulating me on the birth of my son. She was amazed and then seemed annoyed, as she had not been told of all the complications of the birth until she opened my file. Normally she said she did not expect to be told about the actual birth but she said obviously with my problems she should have been informed the next day and naturally she would have seen me on the postnatal ward. I went on to tell her about my couple of problems, the perianal tears and mastitis, but said generally I was fine. When asked about any discharge I mentioned that I had been bleeding regularly but presumed it was normal. Upon this information she examined my stomach, looked concerned and said she had to give me another internal examination. On doing so she exclaimed that she would have to send me back to the main hospital for surgery as the neck of my womb was still wide open. Apparently by this stage it should have closed back to pre-birth size but for some reason mine had not. She commented that I had been incredibly lucky not to have suffered tremendous infection. I remember thinking that it was just as well Nick and I had not been passionate since Dominic was born. Somehow neither of us felt that way inclined.

Feeling relatively lucky about a missed infection I asked when the appointment would be.

'Now,' she replied. 'Today. My dear, this is serious and you need immediate attention. Go home. Pack an overnight bag and go back to the labour ward. I shall phone now to arrange it. You need to go to theatre for them to clean you out properly and tidy you up.'

I was shocked and muttered something about having to breast-feed Dominic. She told me that was not a problem and to take him with me. I returned home in a stunned daze and told an even more stunned Nick. I briefly phoned my mother, packed and off we went.

It seemed very strange to go to the labour ward with a baby! We were a novelty to the staff too who were not used to a baby of six weeks old. I asked their advice about a few things, mainly sleep patterns, but they did not know as it was beyond their experience. I was disappointed that neither of my two favourite midwives were on duty. When we arrived we had to wait for ages in the lounge area. It was a fairly dismal room with a few chairs and a small television plus a few tatty magazines. Nick seemed very edgy, uncomfortable and tired. The whole ward seemed very quiet, deserted almost, so we could not understand the delay and no one told us anything. Eventually I was shown to one of the small side rooms. It was the same one where the doctor had shocked me with his abrupt internal examination when I had been admitted as an emergency. I unpacked and I suggested Nick went home as there was nothing he could do and I would feel better if he went home for a rest.

The midwife said she could look after Dominic whilst I went to theatre. I fed and changed him then got myself ready in the gown. I walked down to the theatre trying to keep the back of my gown together and greeted the masked and appropriately dressed medical team. It brought back memories of the birth, ones I wanted to forget. Then the scratch of the needle, coldness moving up my arm, counting, fading and blackness – but at least it was deep sleep.

When I awoke back in the little room again, guess who needed feeding? Was there never any rest for me? At least this time I did not feel too bad in any way and quite soon I was pottering around the room. Nick came back briefly but again I told him to go and enjoy an undisturbed night. We had to stay the night and once again I spent a couple of hours sleeping but mainly feeding Dominic, changing him and trying as many ways as I could to settle him in the confines of that room. At least the staff popped in every now and then and kept my spirits up with drinks and a chat. They all commented that Dominic was cute and very alert. In the morning I was told I could go home so I phoned Nick to come for us. A midwife offered to entertain the baby whilst I had a shower and got myself ready. When Nick arrived we were both spruced up, feeling fine and we decided to go into Chester, one of our favourite cities.

The phone in the labour ward was not reliable so we had not let my mother know that everything was all right that day. Hours later she had phoned herself to be told we had left before lunchtime. I felt really guilty for having caused her a great deal of unnecessary worry. At least mobile phones now can help alleviate such concerns. Meanwhile we had a successful trip around Chester, managing to have lunch in our favourite café and a mooch in some shops. In Mothercare we put Dominic in a baby walker and Nick took a photograph of him in the display. I presume it was in jest that he said he was up for sale to any offers!

The end of that week was quite happy and we visited Croxteth Park; looked around for a new car; had a barbecue at my parents and had a walk around a local priory. We were getting used to the pram routine and established how it fitted best in the boot. I found life easier with Nick around and thought maybe everything was beginning to settle down. Generally Dominic had now started to go to sleep at night in his crib, occasionally sucking his fists. He could also lift his head up for a few minutes, using his forearms for support if lying on his front. A couple of nights he had slept from 10 p.m. to 3 a.m., which at that time was a huge improvement! He also stayed awake longer in the car and was more alert and responsive. He had a Klippan 'carrytot' seat for the car and although he did not like being put into it, once swung a little he would settle and liked the motion in the car. At least he travelled well.

As Nick had to go back to work I decided to plan a day for Dominic and me, so we went to Altrincham. I found a designer clothes shop which was closing down and bought a huge stock of baby and toddler boy's items for 20% of their original price. I was delighted! He had even behaved on the trip. As a child I had loved trips for clothes and usually got a new dress each season or holiday. My mother always took great pride in dressing us well and I had inherited her desire. Everyday I looked forward to dressing him. During his first summer I favoured the all-in-one romper suits, mainly in white or pale blue. He had been given some cute knee length socks and I used these to finish off the outfit. I also had a huge supply of white cardigans. As he grew I enjoyed hanging up the next size of outfits and packed away his outgrown sets with a smile and hopeful thought of another son (or daughter), wanting to keep everything 'just in case'.

We went to the Mums and Tots group with Sue and Ben as our Tuesday trip and I liked chatting to other mothers. I was faced by surprised looks when I said that Dominic never slept for longer than four hours at a time. His feeding also remained irregular. The next day, having fully prepared him to go out, I decided to walk into town, about half an hour away, for my antenatal class reunion. After ten minutes he was hungry again! I debated what to do and found a tree by the path, sat under it and fed him. My favourite mother and baby changing rooms were at Boots, Mothercare and Safeway. This was a slightly unusual one! At least it gave a few passers-by something to smile about and then we were able to carry on. I chose to walk as much as I could to try to get my weight down. All this feeding made me feel even more indispensable to him. At the class reunion it was lovely to see all the other new babies. I felt very conscious that the other six mums there told their birth stories as if they had read them from the magazines. I glossed over mine. They chatted about their own check-ups which had all be fine; then I told them about mine. Most of the babies already slept through the night and for hours each day. They were a pleasant group of ladies though and we decided to meet up soon at one of our houses. I felt pretty hopeless as we walked back. Why did I seem to complicate everything?

At his six-week check-up, our GP said Dominic was fine and that he was a very alert and intelligent child. This cheered me up a little but still there seemed no end to his demands. However, other compensations that week helped; he made his first definite smiles to us and held a rattle for 20 minutes in his cot. I even managed an hour or two sunbathing on a hot afternoon and felt great relief when he slept all one night with just one short feed at 3 a.m. We had two successful barbecues with family and friends. It was Nick's first Father's Day and he had received his first appropriate card. I was not too sure that he was delighted at this point about being a Dad but I was more optimistic that life would surely begin to be a little easier. I was worried though about my grandmother, following a visit to see the specialist regarding the cancerous growth on her head. The infection had gone but it was not healing up and she would need a skin graft.

On the 17 June it was our first wedding anniversary. Nick was at work so I had a lazy day with Dominic and did bits of beauty treatment in between seeing to him. Mum looked after Dominic whilst Nick and I went for a special meal at a hotel in a local small town called Frodsham. I managed to fit into a white top (with a well-padded bra to hide any leaks!)

and a navy skirt which was too big for me pre-pregnancy. I put it on but had to fasten the top with a large nappy pin as the button and its hole refused to meet! That meant I needed a short-sleeved cardigan over the top to hide it all. I was still twelve pounds heavier than before I had got pregnant. I did think my hair was quite shiny and fell just right, and I enjoyed putting make-up on. I guess I was as human as I could be. We had a romantic evening and talked about our wedding. Was it only 12 months ago? It seemed like a lifetime! We discussed Dominic a little but had decided this was our time together without him for once. The more I ate the tighter the nappy pin became and as the hours wore on I felt my breasts getting heavier and harder. We both agreed that we were glad to be married to each other and although life was proving a challenge at that moment, we convinced ourselves that we were a good team and we would work our way through it together.

The next day I took Dominic into school to show him off to the rest of the staff beyond my class. I was really pleased to be the 'Mum' for once. In my career I seemed to have witnessed this event for so many other staff with new babies and now, at last, it was my turn to see my child being passed around. Nick appeared briefly and left the females to coo, cuddle and gush appropriately. Everyone commented that I looked well and reminded me that September would soon be here and that I should make the most of my time away. A couple of people asked who would be looking after Dominic, an issue still to be sorted. Originally my friend Sue, as a registered child-minder, had said that she would have him. She was now also pregnant with her second child, but as she knew other suitable ladies I was not worried about it.

Later that night we went to see the vicar at the local church to enquire about christenings. Although neither of us had strong religious feelings we believed that the ethos surrounding the church is basically good. We wanted to introduce our child to Christian principles and let him make his own judgements later in life. We both liked the vicar. He was about Nick's age, a former teacher with a very modern outlook. The local primary school was linked to the church and we aimed to send Dominic there when the time came. It made sense to begin links within the parish. Also we knew few people immediately in our area and we thought we might make some new friends too. Ray, the vicar, told me about the new Monday coffee mornings in the church hall and I said I would love to go. We started as we meant to go on and went up to the church fair that weekend.

Another of my friends, Diane, came to see us that weekend. We had first met as volunteers on a holiday for learning disabled teenagers when I was at college. She was taking a year off after her 'A' levels before going into teaching. I recommended my college to her and she followed me there. When she qualified and went to teach I suggested she joined a local Rotaract club. She met her husband, Jon, there and Nick and I were guests at their wedding. She is the sort of friend that even if we do not see each other for months it makes no difference as we just start off from where we left off. Dominic was reasonably settled during their visit and I think they thought our tales of pacing the floorboards with him in the early hours were exaggerated. If only they had been! I now found myself to be cautious in telling couples without children too much detail about pregnancy, birth and life with a newborn, for fear of putting them off. I remember being shocked in the past by other parents who did moan about sleepless nights and decided they were just not doing it right! How judgemental and right-eous I had been, but I was now learning my lesson.

Around this time Nick tried a whole variety of techniques to settle his son, such as playing the piano and putting him on the mini trampoline and bouncing him on it! He often looked quite at a loss as to how to pacify him. I was guilty sometimes of just taking Dominic from him with the easiest answer of feeding him. That must have added even more to Nick's feelings of uselessness. We still tolerated the bath-time routine which proved stressful at times due to Dominic's screams. We had established that Dominic's main cries were hunger, wind, tired or bored. If you could solve these then he may settle and be quiet and content. Often it was hard to solve though.

I found some support at two new groups Dominic and I went to. We began going to the church on Monday mornings where we made friends with another Sue (Sue C from now on) who had a little girl called Sophie. She was four months older than Dominic. Sue was a graduate, like me, and had taken a five-year career break from a good job with a large chemical company. We immediately took to each other and another friendship began. There were some older ladies there who ran many things for the church and it was good to hear their tales and experiences of their own child-rearing years. On a Monday afternoon we also went to a different church group recommended by my other friend Sue. Again it was good to swap stories and tips.

Dominic had a few reasonable nights' sleep, only waking once, so I decided to make my first big trip. My grandfather still had two sisters living at the Fylde coast, Annie (90) and Betty (77). Both were widows and lived alone. They were very lively, capable and good company. Although I had lost touch with my friends from Fleetwood, I always liked to see my great-aunts and naturally wanted to take Dominic to see them. I took my grand-parents too for the day. My grandfather was thrilled to walk his great-grandson along the promenade at his beloved home town – they had moved to Runcorn a few years earlier to be near us all. Dominic was well behaved and found Annie and Betty very interesting. I took some photo-graphs of him with all his eldest relatives and the one of him with his great-grandfather has taken centre place on their fireplace ever since. It was a happy and successful day. My mother had worried that I had taken on too much by doing it but I tried to reassure her that it had indeed been a pleasure and had given me some confidence too. I used to do such trips pre-Dominic, so what was the difference now?

So his two-month stage was marked by this achievement for me. He now weighed 13 lbs 9 oz and was 59 cm long. Generally he would go to bed at 9 p.m., wake at 3 a.m. and 6 a.m., then sleep until 9 a.m. His feeding pattern was varied but feeds were now shorter, ten minutes maximum. He looked much fatter and his hair was regrowing on the top of his head (he had lost some within a couple of weeks of his birth). He had developed a new high-pitched scream if really upset and we could identify some slight differences between other cries. He would respond to me by looking intently at my face and sometimes smile. He often would anticipate a feed. He had begun also to stare at Nick's face and give him a smile. Nick had become the best 'winder' and had more success now rocking and nursing his son. Maybe we were at last becoming a happier family.

CHAPTER 7

We're going to the Lake District

Dominic's third month began with his immunisations. I had received a letter informing me of the time and date at our health centre. I went along presuming it was just us, but no, there seemed to be a surgery full of babies and toddlers, all of whom had been given the same time. We had to line up in the order of arrival outside the nurse's room where the GP was waiting with the relevant jabs. I think the parents looked more worried than the innocent children and bit-by-bit my heart sank as each quiet child or baby came out howling. I had to hold his leg very still while he was 'stabbed'. For the first time as a mother I really wanted the pain to be mine instead of my child's. However, he was fine. It was me who felt a nervous wreck and I am not usually bothered by needles.

He slept well that night and we were both enjoying the luxury of a lie-in, only to be disturbed by someone ringing the door bell every few seconds the next morning. The frequency and intensity was so strong that I panicked that there must be an emergency – could it be a neighbour in trouble? No, just a religious group, yet again, asking me what I thought about the state of the world. They got a very rude and short reply. I was not pleased. I calmed down enough to go to the baby clinic that afternoon and chatted to our health visitor. I told her how pleased I was now with all his energetic kicking and his swings at his play gym and octopus toy each evening. We both hoped such energy would help him to sleep better. He was now tracking objects with his eyes too.

The following day I could not settle Dominic at all. Nothing seemed right, no matter what I tried. By the time Nick came in from school I was almost in tears. Our baby eventually settled down but was very restless and noisy even when asleep. Next day he was worse so we phoned the surgery for advice. As it was Saturday evening we were told a doctor would come from the general support team offered to all the surgeries at such times. At last a doctor arrived but we could hardly understand his accent. He examined Dominic and we made out that he thought it was due to pain in his left thigh due to his injection. A hard lump had formed at the site of the injection. He recommended a drawing ointment, bandages and liquid para-cetamol. We already had the wonderful 'pink drink' in stock but had not yet used any. The doctor advised using a small syringe in the corner of his mouth, so we tried it. Eventually, after a struggle, we succeeded in getting him to take a few drops. It must have been strange for Dominic as all he had drunk so far was my milk. It did settle him for the night though.

Next morning Nick duly applied the drawing ointment, which he had been to collect, and wrapped a bandage around the sore leg, with more struggles. My parents sensed we had been having a trying time and suggested that they looked after Dominic for a few hours. We all had a meal at their house and then we left the baby whilst we relaxed at the cinema. In our absence he had been fine but when we arrived back I had it on my agenda that he had to have more medicine. My parents witnessed us both trying to give him it with a similar fight again. They were mortified that the calm, happy baby they had been looking after was now a distressed, agitated soul and I was cringing that he was making us look like the pathetic, useless parents we were! Oh dear. Within minutes Dominic was dreadfully sick everywhere. We went home.

In the morning I walked up to the church with him and although I noted that Dominic had several smiles for people, for the first time I acknowledged that I felt very low. Later in the day I was back at the health centre for my check-up and other than my mood and general lack of sleep, I felt okay. Physically the GP agreed and I asked if I could resume my aerobic classes which I used to go to before I had Dominic. I got the all clear and that evening I was back at the church hall jumping around! The class teacher really motivated us – a very mixed selection of local ladies of all ages and abilities. It did lift my spirits, although I struggled to keep up. At least it was a start, I told myself. The GP also had looked at Dominic's leg and dismissed the drawing ointment remedy as ridiculous!

That week we also made new acquaintances through Sue C and Sophie. They had joined the NCT group in Frodsham and regularly went to coffee mornings at each other's homes. The four of us went and I was introduced to yet another group of new mothers, mostly with careers that they intended to go back to. Once again I found I seemed to be the only one with a child of Dominic's age who was not sleeping at night. Surely it was not just us? Were other people afraid to say they had bad times too? Everyone else appeared so capable and one lady was already expecting her second child when her first was not much older than mine! The nearest we got to intimacy or sex in our house was a cup of coffee at the same time! Later that day we called to see another friend of mine who had a son a year older than mine. I would never, ever want to wish difficulties on any parents but what a relief it was to hear that they too had problems – for example, their child refused to settle down for ages at bedtime! At least now we had one saving grace as Dominic, who had become addicted to his thumb, would soon drift off to sleep (even if not for long). This further convinced me that all the other parents, whom I did not know that well, were possibly not being so generous with the truth, yet my good friends did not mind being totally honest. Such thought processes refuelled my enthusiasm for parenthood again and I fought on with renewed optimism.

That weekend we had booked for Claire and us to spend two nights in a small hotel near Coniston, in the Lake District. I think we must have decided to do this during a brief, good moment! The rooms were tiny, with very thin walls, which immediately concerned us. If Dominic woke during the night he would disturb many people! Claire was really impressed by how much her nephew had grown and was fascinated by his responsiveness. We had planned to dine at the hotel that evening but were informed by the management that a baby would not be welcome. What were we supposed to do with him? Leave him in a wardrobe? Undaunted, I searched through my guide of pubs and restaurants which welcomed children. Relief was felt all round when I found a reference to a place in Ambleside which was very child-friendly, with good baby-changing and feeding facilities. We phoned, explained we had a 10-week-old baby and would it be acceptable for us all to dine there that evening. They were happy to accept our booking so we then went for a walk in a small area called 'The Hawk'. I enjoyed seeing Claire and kept her up to date with recent happenings and Dominic seemed to like the fresh air. Typically he needed refreshment en route.

We all returned to the hotel and got changed. I had my navy skirt on again. This time without the nappy pin holding it together, but it was still tight. I wanted a really good photograph of us as a family and Claire took a selection. We both looked shattered on them and Dominic was just not trained yet as a model! We did get some cute ones of him with his auntie though. On to Ambleside where we were given a table with a big bench seat so I could have some room for the baby and all his equipment. We ordered our meals which were rather exotic and much more expensive than in the guide. We had anticipated steak and chips, instead a new chef was creating very fancy and rich cordon bleu delights. I sought out the ladies' toilet where indeed there was a chair suitable for feeding. It was his usual bed and drink time but he fought with me and refused to take any. After a while I returned to the table where Nick and Claire had been staring at their starters, waiting for me. I had one mouthful and Dominic started to cry. By now the restaurant had begun to fill up with couples for a romantic night out, candles and wine on the tables. I paced the street for a while with him to no avail. I returned to eat mine whilst Nick retreated outside. Before the main course came I tried to feed him again and he had a little but still refused to settle.

We had to eat our main course in shifts again and all three of us attempted different ways to get him to sleep. I had to change him once more and he took a little more milk. I tried gripe water. I tried playing. Two couples asked to be moved from near our table (who could blame them!) and others looked on sympathetically. I kept apologising to the waitress and explained we had used the guide, not expecting the restaurant to be such a swish Saturday night venue. She said that they did not even know they were in such a guide and did not blame us for being misled. Why did he settle so well every night at home and not for us now? I had anticipated giving him his feed and then he would have drifted off to sleep, lulled by the mellow jazz music, chatter and candlelight. Yes, I was wrong again. All we succeeded in doing was getting indigestion and a big bill and adding to our stress levels as parents. I felt sorry for Claire too who described the evening, years later, as a 'nightmare'. These days I realise how overambitious we were and know to cut our losses at the first sign of an unsuitable menu and ambience and eat fish and chips on a bench in the street!

Of course as soon as we got in the car, Dominic nodded off to sleep blissfully. I think we were all tempted to poke him awake then for spoiling our evening. We got him up to the room without a peep, got into the small, lumpy double bed and muttered about the evening. Just as we were going to sleep, he woke up. After another proper feed and change he settled by midnight, but I lay awake waiting for him to wake up again. Relaxation was not in my system. I do not think Nick had much sleep either. Neither of us had anywhere to escape to. Sometimes just knowing you can go to another room helps you to relax. We were very conscious of disturbing the neighbours too. Amazingly we got through the small hours with him asleep but then had a struggle between five and six in the morning. At breakfast time all of us were fast asleep and then only just made it down in time for last orders! Typical!

We soon packed up and vowed to try to make a success of something about the trip. It began to rain but undeterred we drove to Tarn Hows and walked around the water. Somehow getting back into nature is soothing. The sounds of birds and water are always calming and the very gentle rain combined to help ease our exhaustion and exasperations. I think I admitted to Claire that motherhood was proving much harder than I had ever imagined and wondered how single parents cope. Although the strain was beginning to show on Nick and I, there was never a moment when I wished our baby was not around. Halfway along our walk the rain stopped. I took Dominic out of his pram for more photographs. I look even more exhausted! We carried on to a craft shop and tearoom for a light lunch then looked around the shops in Keswick. Both Nick and I enjoyed walking so when we spotted a papoose for babies and small toddlers we wanted it. It was like a rucksack but had a seat for the child instead, who was supposed to enjoy being carried in it once they had head control. We even bought the accessory bag, sun and rain shades to go with it as we intended to do plenty of walking that summer as part of our 'normal' (what was that?) lifestyle. It appeared to brighten up Nick's mood and after a successful meal in a lively, bustling cafe, Claire returned to Glasgow and we came home. At least Dominic was content on the journey back.

Once at home he settled quickly in his crib again, sucking his thumb, waking at two-hourly intervals from 2.30 a.m. I had always thought that fresh air tired you out, but not this child. A day or two later I was back at the doctors' surgery with mastitis again and had to have more antibiotics. Then we had to take the pram-base back to the shop as it had collapsed on me and would not click back into place. They lent me a temporary replacement. Even this ended up as a problem later in the week. I took my grandparents shopping with me and when we were loading up the car to go back, the pram chassis jammed onto the base and would not budge! Dominic began screaming because the car had not begun to move, my grandfather no longer had the strength in his hands to help and my grandmother did not seem to realise there was a problem. As my tears began, a kind gentleman in the car park came to my aid and saved the day.

Meanwhile I went to all my group meetings that week and felt so inadequate amongst all these other mothers who appeared to cope with everything. I hosted our first antenatal coffee afternoon. Luckily Dominic was a model child and a couple of the others admitted to a few hiccups too. He even had a happy bath time with his father that night. In retrospect I had come to feel I was on a roller coaster, as just as I found it all too much then something good would happen and reinstate my optimism and confidence to plod on. Dominic had begun to smile much more and even make a few sounds instead of cries. Physically he was doing well and now could raise both his legs together when on his back.

I had used his cot in the nursery as a safe place to lie him down and sometimes change him. At times he was content to lie in it and watch his mobile and knock his toys whilst I pottered upstairs. That weekend was another step forward as I left him to nap in it. All along I had the aim for him to be sleeping well in his own cot at night for when I went back to work full time in September. He would use a bottle to have a drink of water . from other people and although I was never able to use a breast pump, I used some small breast shells to collect bits of milk for others to give him if I was not there. I found that I leaked so much from one breast whilst he was sucking on the other that it made sense to pop one of these little shaped tubs in my bra and collect milk at the same time. As the school summer holidays were approaching, it reminded me of the impending return to work and I had to try to make weaning progress with him too. I kept wondering how I would survive on all this irregular broken sleep and work as well, but convinced myself that everything would be fine.

Nick and I went shopping into Liverpool one day and decided to appreciate the sunshine on the way home with a walk along Otterspool Promenade, at the side of the River Mersey. It turned out to be a serious 'heart-to-heart' discussion. Nick began by asking when would Dominic talk and walk. He admitted how hard he was finding everything, a disappointment really, due to the complete disruption to our lives. The tiredness was the main factor but he just could not see the happiness factor to be gained when we were putting in so much hard work to see so little reward. Out of every 24 hours we might get a couple of reasonable ones. He summed up by stating, 'I just want him to grow up.'

Of course initially I felt upset. My image of a husband being so besotted with our child and thus loving me even more for my part in creating it just evaporated. I had longed so much for the picture that is seen so often of the handsome couple gazing blissfully down at their sleeping child. What had I done wrong? Why wasn't it like this? I seemed to hear so many other mothers saying how devoted their husbands or partners were with their babies, so it must be my fault. My own father was fabulous with newborn babies and youngsters in general. I also did realise that there were many other fathers who did not bond with their youngsters until they were older and again convinced myself that his love for Dominic would grow in time. He mentioned the birth. Having been left holding this newborn 'creature' who had caused his wife so much pain, and seeing her being rushed off for surgery in pools of blood as a result, did not get them off to a good start. Since then all he had witnessed was me being ill, exhausted and never relaxing; little time to ourselves and all our usual pleasures curtailed in some way.

I was unable to disagree with him and although disappointed by his comments I also understood them. He was right about it all. After living on his own for years he had made many compromises when it was just the two of us and we had only just settled to those. Now we had a child and every notion of normality had disappeared and I suppose he feared the woman he had married had also gone. After yearning for a child all my life, I equally did not want anything to spoil my current feeling of fulfilment and joy at finally achieving it. I accepted that Dominic was very, very demanding and that I also was shocked and worried by the almighty effect he had had upon our lives. I expressed my pleasure at this stage of his life in spite of the seemingly endless tasks he demanded of me. I appealed to Nick to be patient, that one day of course our child would walk and talk, but in the meantime asked him to bear with me and not spoil these precious months for me.

We agreed to differ in our current aspirations. If I could cope with his apprehension then he would try to handle my overenthusiasm. In the meantime, what should we do? I agreed that I should let others do more for Dominic and not be so possessive of him. I tried to explain that I felt that as my time with him at home was only a few more months then I wanted to do it all. I was not being a martyr. We tried to think what used to make us happy and decided that mutual exercise was something and hence attempted to commit to get fit. Our leisure club membership had lapsed so we decided to go back and swim together. People often left babies at the side of the pool in their car seats. Almost with a smile we realised that if other babies did it then Dominic would not! Instead we agreed that one would attend to him whilst the other swam. No matter what, we were still both glad to be together and vowed to persevere. Nick could see I was getting increasingly down and tired in reality. I was blind to it because I was still on such a high and wanted everything to be perfect.

The following afternoon we both managed a swim and then left Dominic with his grandparents for a few hours while we had time to ourselves. I joined my hospital friend Jeannie at her antenatal class reunion in Chester. Dominic cried a lot. Then another sleepless night as his first cold developed. I had three very trying days with him due to his cold. I had become very skilled in making up excuses for him and not asking for help. In the midst of his screams on one of those days my head teacher came for a social visit and to chat to me about coming back to work in September. I attempted to convince her and myself that all would be well then. This was just a minor hiccup.

After a few days I insisted we were both fine and had another Fleetwood trip with the elderly relatives. 'Of course I was not tired' and 'I was going because I wanted to', I told mother and Nick, who were not impressed. My time at home was running out for such things so I had to make the most of it. It was another successful day out that we all enjoyed. Yet Dominic then screamed on and off all night, making me cringe that he was giving Nick evidence to prove we should not have gone. Why did this child seem to make everything so awkward? No wonder Nick was finding it hard, as he thrives on routine and this child created a new one every day. Even shopping for food was a challenge that week. I had begun to successfully judge when I could attempt it and Dominic was beginning to be quite content playing with a toy or crinkly bit of paper in the trolley. This week he was not and could be heard throughout the store! Full marks to the Safeway store as one member of staff pushed my trolley for me whilst I held him, another unloaded it at the till and repacked it, then another put it all in the car for me!

Additional stress was again balanced by a sociable, sunny weekend with more barbecues with family and friends. Plenty of red wine helped too. Even I indulged, having been teetotal as a pregnant and then breast-feeding mother. We all decided it might make Dominic sleep! They all commented on how well he was doing. He could now use two hands together and explore objects with his mouth. His party piece was now his smiles for most people. The trail of presents still continued from various people and rekindled my excitement again. When we were in company, Dominic usually shone and almost made me feel like a liar for complaining about how demanding he was. People would say things like 'All babies settle in time', 'He's a pretty little baby', 'He's well behaved when he's awake; he's very alert, very, very bright', 'Oh, he's gorgeous! What's the matter with you? You've got everything you always wanted now'. I learnt not to complain.

As my final week off in term time approached I was determined to fill it positively. Dominic and I went to our church groups. We invited Sue and Ben to visit us one afternoon. Sue was six months pregnant and struggling in the heat. I had to take him for his next injections and he cried loudly. I took him and my grandparents shopping and went out with my mother too. One evening I asked Nick to keep an eye on our baby whilst I did something. I looked out of the window a while later to see him with Dominic contentedly on his back in the papoose, whilst he got on with watering the bedding plants! We were all busy, busy, busy.

On the penultimate morning of the summer term at school, Nick was woken by me sobbing at 6 a.m. I suddenly had panicked about my return to work. I felt I really would not be able to cope with everything that being a working mother would entail. I was useless at this baby thing. I was failing as a wife, so how on earth could I be a good teacher too? He was very good listening to me as I wailed and in the end must have succeeded in calming me down before he faced his day at work. My mother also reassured me later that everything would be fine and we went into Liverpool for our lunch. My last day 'off' before the school holidays was spent at a beautiful house in Manley at an NCT coffee morning with Sue C and Sophie. Later I attended our Leavers Assembly at school for those from my class who were 19 and off to pastures new. Everyone commented that it would be good to see me back after the holidays and thus my maternity leave ended, hence resuming full pay – phew!

As Dominic approached three months old I was rather frazzled but he now weighed 14 lbs 12 oz and was 61.5 cm long. Generally he would go to bed at 8.30 p.m., wake at 2 a.m. and 5 a.m., then sleep until 8.30 a.m. His feeding pattern was varied but feeds continued to be shorter – at ten minutes maximum. He looked much fatter and had improved his head control. He could bring his hands together, turn to sounds, and suck his thumb and fingers. He had developed a range of happy sounds and would 'talk' to us.

Yes, just maybe, progress was being made.

CHAPTER 8

A holiday

Nick and I left Dominic with my parents one night whilst we went up to the vicarage to attend a christening meeting. At our church they held the actual christenings monthly at a special afternoon service and would have about four to six youngsters involved at the same time. That evening meeting was for those intending to have their service on the first Sunday in September. Ray discussed various issues surrounding the service and the church in general. We thought this would be a good time for Dominic's christening as it would be the day before we went back to work. This happy event followed by a meal for our closest family and friends would be ideal. The arrangements were duly made and I felt pleased about them. We had decided to ask Roy, Nick's college friend, to be his godfather, with Claire and Sue (Ben's mother) as godmothers.

On the first day of the summer holidays we stripped the big back bedroom ready to decorate it. We went and chose a carpet and ordered a bed settee. As we rarely had guests staying overnight we decided that a single pine bed with another 'hidden' underneath would be a good use of space and as Dominic grew then it would become his playroom. The small front bedroom was fine for a nursery and subsequent bedroom but not very big for all his toys and equipment in the future. Nick and I thrive on having 'a project' and the planning for this room and subsequent actions were beginning to make us both feel better. Dominic spent his first night sleeping in his cot in the nursery, another step forward. I kept checking on him with a paintbrush in my hand as we had decided to start the window frame!

The nursery and 'blue room' are opposite each other at the front of the house. With Dominic now in the nursery, we decided Nick would sleep in our bedroom again and I would be in the blue room if needed by Dominic. That first night I was up at 12.30 a.m. (just as I had gone to sleep), then again at 5 a.m. The following day he suffered from wind and even screamed at his grandparents. I had to abandon the painting in order to try to pacify him. We persevered with him in the cot, which was more successful the next few nights.

For Nick's birthday that week we had a barbeque for our friends and families. We also started Dominic on his first few spoons of baby rice. Plenty of people had advised me that once he started on solids he would sleep better. He did not like it and screamed. He had to have it as far as I was concerned and even attempted it whilst our guests were with us, silly me. I then had to contend with everyone's well meant but contradictory advice, leaving me once again feeling useless as a mother. I wonder now why I was so tough on myself. In retrospect I realise I was getting far too hung up about such matters instead of leaving them until another time. I seemed to be developing such impatience and urgency. This may have been due to the underlying worry of going back to work.

His first week on solids developed from one teaspoon of baby rice each evening, ranging from him taking it quite happily to screaming, with us debating each time about the consistency, his position and various other factors. By the fifth day, when I was still struggling, I phoned Sue for advice. The following two nights were great with him smiling and kicking his legs, so we progressed to two spoonfuls! This happened to be on my 33rd birthday – the first anniversary of my baby being conceived. I was really happy that day and felt satisfied that in my grand plan of life I had finally made it to motherhood, albeit five years later than anticipated. We began the day with a family attendance at communion at church where we were made most welcome. We sat near the back in case Dominic was a problem but he was reasonably good. Later my parents and Claire called with presents. My parents gave me a beautiful white china figurine of a mother and baby. I loved it. As it was a sunny day we decided to go to Cholmondley Castle Gardens for a walk and afternoon tea. The backdrop of the foliage was perfect for more photographs and I still beamed with pride and contentment. Back home we treated ourselves to a steak, strawberries and champagne meal, interrupted by Dominic's cries.

The next week I began arranging the christening properly by ordering a cake and sending out invitations. Dominic's diet evolved further to tastes of fruit and vegetables plus the baby rice twice a day. Farley's rusks went down well. They used to be my favourite. Naturally I had read all the books and magazines again for this stage and had stocked up on tiny dishes to make and freeze meals for him. Meanwhile we had finished decorating the back bedroom; had workmen in for a couple of days who ripped out and replaced the downstairs shower room; then Nick began painting the hall and stairs! This was supposed to be holiday time!

I went for my first real night out with some girls for my friend Debbie's hen night. We went for a Greek meal on the outskirts of Manchester. Debbie had adored Greek food since she and I had a fabulous holiday together in Zakynthos two years earlier. I was delighted that she was getting married but I did not really enjoy the night. I realised how tired I was. I felt frumpy and fat. I did not know any of the other guests and I just wanted to go to bed. It dawned on me that I had entered the realms of being a boring mother. What had happened to the fun-loving, flirty, attention-seeking partygoer from that Greek holiday? She felt 20 years older and her breasts hurt. I occasionally thought of Dominic and the changes in him recently. He was holding his head up more, smiled at himself in the mirror, rolled onto his side and could move his body around by kicking. Nick actually put his son to bed for the first time that evening and all went well for them. We had started him on some formula milk too as part of the weaning process and he had taken to it well.

We continued to attend the various church and antenatal group coffee mornings and afternoons, leaving Nick to enjoy his household chores and decorating. I managed to find a dress that fitted me for Debbie's wedding that weekend. I still could not wear my previous clothes and trying them on had depressed me. I had been going to aerobics on Mondays and was at last beginning to keep up with the pace. Each week I could do a bit more and I really switched off from all my concerns as I concentrated on the exercises. However, it was not enough yet to slip back into a size 12. In the past I had liked myself with curly, permed hair so I thought if I went back to this it might lift my spirits. Richard was not keen to do it as he said that look was dated and my current sleek bob was great. I could not be convinced and so it was duly permed. It did not take well (probably due to the chemical changes in my body) and I was left with a tatty, unkempt look that I did not want! Oh dear again! I compensated for my hair disappointment by giving Dominic his first meal sitting in his high chair. He did enjoy food and I liked watching his reactions to new tastes.

All three of us went to Debbie and Alan's wedding. I had been reluctant to take the baby but she said there would be others going too and not to worry. He wore a white and navy velour suit which felt so cuddly. Dominic was now quite a chubby little baby and I could not cuddle him enough, especially when he was wearing something so tactile. Our relaxation was thin on the ground though as throughout the service and speeches we had to try incredibly hard to keep him quiet and amused. He liked to pull my hat and Nick looked very much the new father, wearing his suit with a white cloth over his shoulder! It was really nice to see Debbie so happy and she looked stunning in the dress we had chosen together whilst I was pregnant. The weather was perfect and at the reception the photographer busily organised groups of appropriate people. It was a lovely wedding, but I did not relax and felt very, very tired.

We called to see Nick's mother on the way home. She was thrilled to see us and as usual had more gifts for her grandson. She had begun to hold him now he was a bit bigger and today he chuckled at her beautifully. Yet again a high followed a low. We returned to the evening reception without him. I used to love dancing, but although the music was good I just did not feel like joining in. The next day we went to a christening at Chester, for Jeannie's son Oliver. After the service there was an excellent buffet at their home and we all spilled out into the garden due to the heatwave. There were several people I knew from her antenatal group and we were introduced to members of her family, but I found myself struggling to chat. I used to be a very sociable person and could talk to anyone. Over this weekend I had begun to feel socially inept. I did not know what to say to people. I felt irritable and snappy. If anyone paid me a compliment I almost wanted to accuse them of lying. There was nothing currently good about me.

Next morning the three of us went to see my parents about looking after Dominic from September, as they had originally offered to and we wanted to confirm it. Neither of us had ever wanted them to have to have him on a regular basis. I believed grandparents should be there for treats and being spoilt, not as a necessity. They had looked after us three for years and they did not deserve to be tied down with a demanding baby. Other people had commented that youngsters who spent a great deal of time with grandparents tended to be more old-fashioned and more clingy. Consequently, when my mother said she had decided to continue as a school librarian, we did not mind. My father was working part time as a first-aid instructor and he said he would be able to have him quite a bit. We were not worried at this stage as Sue had recommended another child-minder. I had met this lady, Cathy, at a church group and we said we would contact her.

Back at home I got Cathy's number and asked her if she could take Dominic full time from September. Her reply stunned me as due to us telling her my parents would be looking after Dominic, she had agreed to take some other children! She could have him two days a week initially though. In a panic I phoned Sue and she tried some other friends who were registered child-minders, but to no avail. Then I remembered that one of the ladies I had talked to at the baby clinic a few times had told me that she was a nursery nurse and since her little boy was born a month before Dominic she had applied for child-minding registration. After a few phone calls I tracked her down, told her my problem and went round to see her. I had to accept that she was not officially registered, but she would include him in everything with her son and she would obviously be pleased with the money we would pay her. Thus settled, I went back home to report to Nick. Later my mother came round and we told her Cathy could have Dominic two days a week so she said that between my father's days off and hers then they would probably manage the other three days. Obviously that would be much cheaper for us and as the other lady's arrangements were complicated I phoned her, thanked her for the offer but explained we no longer needed it. I felt embarrassed and mean at having built her up to let her down.

Feeling reasonably sorted we left the next day for our first family holiday. I had found a cheap hotel offer at Corby in Leicestershire for two nights. When we checked in and went up to our room it was adequate but Nick decided to enquire about an upgrade. A few minutes later he came back with a key for the 'Brampton suite' for an extra £20 a night. It was incredible! We had a huge bathroom, including bidet, a dressing room, massive bedroom plus lounge and dining area. The best bit was its own hall area which bypassed the bedroom and bathroom to the living area. This was ideal for the cot and I made Dominic's 'home' in that area. We had luxury robes, wine and a basket of fruit and sweets too. Brilliant! We had space to spread out and we definitely relaxed and enjoyed the rooms. Nick and I coped in the one huge bed and Dominic only woke once in the night for a quick feed and immediately settled again. He had his first swim in the leisure pool and other bathers commented on how well he had taken to it. We were actually having a good time together at last.

We spent the next day visiting Uppingham, then Oakham, and had a pleasant walk around Rutland Water with Dominic happily kicking his legs in his pram and chatting to his hands. Our meals out were acceptable and we returned back to the hotel for another swim and leisurely night in our suite. It was well worth the extra money. When Dominic woke that night I was able to take him into the lounge area and feed him just using the car park lights and passing headlights to see by. As I sat curled up on the settee with Dominic suckling me, I felt a wave of love for him that I had not really felt before. He was staring up at me, gulping away, then he suddenly stopped, caught my eye and smiled at me. Milk dribbled over both of us but I did not care. He was my baby and I loved him. His smell. His feel. His smile. He had exhausted both Nick and I, but I really thought from now on everything would be fine and that the worst was over. Full and content, Dominic fell asleep on me and I just stayed with him for a little longer. Eventually I tucked him back in the cot and snuggled back in with Nick with a contented sigh.

Next morning we left after breakfast, declaring that at least we had actually had a successful hotel stay, and set off for home. We stopped at Chatsworth House where Dominic attracted a great deal of attention in his papoose. The only place he really objected was in the bulging noisy cafe where we had to queue and then try to find a table. Poor Nick looked so embarrassed as all the diners turned to see the source of the howling child. Once at a table he settled and he later fell asleep in the papoose when we walked around the house. Back at home he had his first night without an early morning feed – hurray!

We entertained Sue, Jon, Jeannie and her husband for a meal (without the babies) and I actually enjoyed cooking and being sociable without feeling it was a great effort. We had also cleaned the house from top to bottom and were proud to show them our new decor and cloakroom. I felt aspects of the 'old me' emerging and felt we were starting to have an acceptable level of family life.

So as Dominic approached four months old I was beginning to get back on an even keel. Generally he would go to bed at 9 p.m., wake at 5 a.m. then sleep until 9.30 a.m. He had three naps in the daytime. He was breast-fed now just at breakfast, late afternoon and bedtime and took a range of pureed foods and formula milk. He could roll onto his side, kick around on his back a full 360 degrees and had better head control. He had developed a range of noises and could chuckle and 'shout'. His favourite activities were knocking the pieces of his gym, talking to his hands, kicking his legs, waving his arms and smiling and talking to people.

Only a few weeks until I went back to work and I thought we had cracked it.

CHAPTER 9

Dominic's in hospital!

After our mini-holiday, generally we were all getting along better. One strength of our marriage was the ability to listen to each other about any problems, usually understand each other's point of view and come to a compromise. The concerns we had expressed to each other earlier in the summer had been improved on and bit by bit, as Dominic was responding more, Nick was likewise responding to him. I think this was the last burst of optimism I felt without then expecting a fall of some kind. Little did we know what was to come.

On August Bank Holiday Monday, Dominic was very sick all day. He had never been a sickly baby so this naturally worried me. We coped by just having a lazy day to tend to him. Next day he had another of his immunisations and seemed better. We went to my parent's for a meal and they gave Dominic a beautiful handcrafted rocking horse as an early Christening present – a definite heirloom. Next day Nick and I left him with them whilst we went shopping and had lunch out in Manchester for a treat. Before Dominic went to bed that night we took many photographs of him using the new soft filter Nick had been given as a birthday present. He was giggling, smiling and looked a very content baby. We had learnt to respond and solve his cries appropriately these days and consequently his cries were fewer and farther apart. He even slept all night for the very first time!

Next morning when he did wake up, he had a very high temperature. He slept again most of the morning but we still went with Sue and Ben to Cathy's for lunch to discuss child-minding arrangements. They reassured me that he probably would soon perk up. Dominic continued to be hot and became very miserable. As it was baby clinic day I decided to take him to seek advice. They reassured me there that it was probably a reaction to the jab a few days earlier and that it was quite common. All day he would not take a bottle or solids so I gave him breast-feeds to comfort and hydrate him. All night he continued to be very hot and sick occasionally, so I put him in the big bed with me as I found it easier than straining at every sound from across the landing. He began to get very listless too with a rash beginning to appear. Feeling very concerned we phoned the 24-hour emergency line for advice and they sent out a locum doctor from an agency. We could just about understand what he said, 'Well, yes, this baby's very poorly, but ring the surgery in the morning.'

The only other thing he said was to keep him warm. This seemed odd when all the books we had consulted before ringing advised the opposite. As new, naive parents you take the doctor's word as gospel and abide by it. The hours seemed to drag until we knew our usual surgery opened its telephone line. As soon as we got through the receptionist told us to bring him in straight away, when I explained the situation. I just grabbed his pram bag (always restocked after every trip) and off we went to our surgery.

We were told to go straight down to the doctor who after a brief look at him and discussion with us, announced, 'This child needs hospitalisation now.'

Before I realised what was going on he asked if we had a car with us. We nodded and he phoned the children's ward at the general hospital, informing them that there was a four-month-old baby on his way with suspected meningitis. He quickly wrote us a letter to give to them on the children's ward and wished us well. I muttered something about nipping home first to get a few things but he insisted that we must not delay at any cost. I wrapped up Dominic again and went back to the car in a daze. Meningitis? No, I told myself, that cannot be right. It was just a reaction to the injection. He would be fine. As Nick drove as fast as he legally (or otherwise) could, I sat in the back staring in disbelief at Dominic. My blood raced through my veins in sheer panic as I realised his pupils were not reacting to changes in light as they usually did. His eyes were flat and dull with huge dilated centres. Dread and horror swept over me as the possible implications of the suspected illness dawned on me. In our teaching careers we had both taught children who had been brain damaged by that very disease. Their deformed little bodies came to mind and as much as I love my pupils I could not help my current fears.

'Please, please God,' I prayed, 'we have both dedicated years to such children. Please, please do not let us end up with one of our own.'

Neither of us spoke on the 20-minute journey.

Nick found the relevant car park and then had to face the ridiculous hassle of finding a pay and display ticket machine! I did not want to go in without him. Our child was critically ill and yet the system demands you add to your worries in this way. Luckily, as an organised couple we always have a bag of change for parking. The GP had given us strict instructions to go straight to a children's ward and not Accident and Emergency. We followed the signs, with me clutching Dominic in a blanket, and I expected the usual request to sit and wait to be seen. As soon as we introduced ourselves at the nurse's station, however, staff appeared from nowhere. We went into a small room with a bed in it and a doctor asked me to strip Dominic down to his nappy, and they examined him whilst he was on my lap. He was still incredibly hot, listless and had a rash. There were a couple of doctors or maybe a consultant plus several nurses; I was not sure. They asked Nick and I about the last few days and they soon decided they needed to put a line into him to take blood and possibly give him a drip. Several staff tried for ages, unsuccessfully, as his veins had collapsed. All the time I was holding him. His little face was contorted with distress. He screamed blue murder. They tried in each arm, each leg, his feet and even his skull. You name it, they tried. I could sense their panic about needing to do it and I was useless to assist. I could take his piercing, unnatural scream no longer and began to cry myself. In the end they had to send me out because I was just getting too distressed.

One aspect which made it worse was that the only serious illness I had as a child was viral meningitis and pneumonia when I was ten. From being fine at lunchtime I had developed a headache, went delirious and was rushed to hospital by early evening, where it took several staff to hold me down for a lumbar puncture. I still remembered the excruciating pain of the headache and confusion of drifting in and out of consciousness. My baby was going through the same and there was nothing I could do to stop it. I had fully recovered. He might not. Still the thought came – how could fate be so cruel? We have helped all these brain-damaged children all these years, and it looks like we might end up with one of our own. I had some change in my pocket and knew what to do. I needed my mother badly. I found a phone in the corridor, dialled and she answered.

'Oh Mum,' I began, and then continued with tears rolling down my cheeks to pour out what had happened. I described in detail about his eyes, the scream, his body heat, the team of staff with him and how scared I was. I wondered why she did not reply, then realised the telephone had not accepted the money and I had been telling only passers-by in the corridor. Why is it that when your emotions are raw you can jump to extremes, like getting the urge to giggle at a funeral? I wanted to laugh hysterically at myself, but at least it jolted me sufficiently to calm down a little, redial and tell the events in a clearer fashion. My poor mother was equally devastated but did her best to hide it and reassure me that it probably was not that serious, and reminding me of her words of wisdom 'worry when something happens and not before'. Feeling a little braver, I made my way back down the corridor to the ward and felt relieved not to hear him screaming.

In the room Dominic now looked swamped on the large bed and there seemed to be drips and wires and monitors everywhere from him. He looked so small on the big expanse of white linen. I know I like a baby in white, but not like this. Nick had stayed with them throughout. The staff now appeared calmer and they explained to us that they were treating him for meningococcal septicaemia and meningitis but we would have to wait for results of the tests. They had taken fluid from his spine and several blood samples. No matter what the outcome they explained that it would be a minimum stay of seven days due to the necessary intravenous antibiotics he needed. They also told us that Nick and I would need to take a precautionary drug to prevent us developing his condition and they warned that it could induce flu-like symptoms in us. Along with the tablets came an A4 sheet describing the possible side-effects. We were told I could stay and that as a breast-feeding mother I would be given my meals free of charge. Dominic would stay in an isolation room on the ward and although we could have visitors they discouraged me from going into other rooms there.

They left the three of us alone for a while. It seemed so very still and quiet after all the commotion, but at least Dominic looked more peaceful. Someone brought us a cup of tea, a small gesture but greatly appreciated, which we drank as we came to terms with the shock of the morning. I do not think either of us could actually believe what had happened and I do not remember saying very much other than we would have to cancel the christening (three days away) and that it looked like I would have at least another week off work. The first few days were training days so I would not be letting anyone down. We asked for some paper and I wrote out a list of things I needed for us both in hospital. Not again! The required items appeared from my memory as easily as a weekly shopping list. We decided that Nick would go home and collect the necessary things, make some phone calls and return later. Before he left I phoned my mother back who said she would be over to see us as soon as possible.

When Nick left I stood at the side of my sleeping baby, stroking his bruised limbs from all the needle attempts. Tears fell again as I tried to make sense of the situation. All I wanted was a husband and family. Why were we being thrown so many problems? Everyone else seemed to sail through it all. Why not us? Was it because I had defied my first marriage vows? Was I being paid back for all of that? Luckily a nurse came in to check on his monitors and observations. She consoled me and told me that hopefully he was over the worst, he was in the best place and they were doing all they could for him. Clichés maybe, but words you need to hear in such circumstances. She passed me a tissue and commented what a beautiful baby he was and I must be proud of him. Kind words mean so much when your world has just been blown apart.

Before long my mother arrived bearing flowers, magazines, goodies and the best things of all – moral support and unconditional love. She too was naturally upset to see her precious grandson attached to wires and drips. Nursing staff and the occasional doctor came in to see Dominic regularly and such attention did make me feel confident that if there was a problem it would be picked up and dealt with. I started my course of tablets and Nick had taken his with him. Soon his sister Glenys appeared with a floating helium balloon and card for her nephew. I felt very touched that she too had rushed over – word had soon spread with Nick telling everyone that the christening was postponed.

The meal trolley appeared at teatime but I declined the offer of some sandwiches as my mother had brought me some treats from Marks and

Spencer. I did not feel hungry, but as the only nutrition they suggested for Dominic for a few days was breast milk I had to keep my intake up. I was able to cuddle him if I stayed right at the side of the bed provided a nurse handed him to and from me. He did have a couple of small feeds that first day but was very listless. How I longed to see him kicking his legs and giggling. Nick returned with all the bags and yet again I 'made home' in a hospital room. It was reasonably big with a couple of armchairs, washbasin and bedside cabinet. The view was just out to a courtyard area with little to watch or see. It was with weary hearts and dismay of the situation that Nick and I said goodnight that evening as I walked with him to the main corridor. I cried bitterly as he walked away and I returned to the bleep of the monitors.

I was provided with a folding bed and linen to put at the side of Dominic's big cot. It was old and there was a huge dent in the middle where it had been folded up. It creaked every time I even moved a finger. The lights from the nurse's station right by the room were dimmed slightly at night but it was all much too light to sleep. My baby had to be checked on and/or given more drugs every two hours, so just as I might be slipping off to sleep a nurse would come in to see to him. It was impossible for them to do this unnoticed so I hardly slept and saw every hour on my watch. I heard every stage of development as a couple of other patients were admitted. I think I settled at around 5 a.m., then just after 6 a.m. ward life begun with the lights going on fully again, noises of staff changing shift and then an auxillary nurse swinging the door open to ask if I wanted a cup of tea! I gave up and got up! Two nights again without sleep. At least Dominic had slept quite well.

After breakfast I washed and got dressed. Leggings and t-shirt plus my slippers were all that was required. Sylvia, Nick's mother, came to see us both and brought some flowers which brightened up the room. She too could hardly believe the situation. I felt guilty that I was in danger of becoming a drama queen – why couldn't I just have a baby and get on quietly like everyone else? The nursing and medical staff continued to be wonderful in every way in attending to both Dominic's and my needs. I asked if I was in the way as a fussing mother as another tiny baby had been brought in during the night and its parents had gone. That child cried most of the time. The nurses assured me that they liked parents to stay because the children were often happier and just being there to comfort them was a huge benefit to all involved. Once again their kind words were a tonic to me.

During the day we had plenty of visitors in addition to Nick – my parents and grandparents, Claire and Glenda, a close colleague of mine, plus Ray the vicar. I was surprised but pleased to see him and not only did he reassure me that another christening could be arranged but he also said a prayer for Dominic lying there. The medical staff were pleased with his progress and gradually all the wires and drips were removed, just leaving a line in one arm. This was a huge relief and we were able to bath him. He cried! Nick is always intrigued by new surroundings and went exploring the ward. He found a room with two beds in it plus an en-suite toilet and shower room. He enquired at the nurse's station who said it was for two children who did not have infectious conditions but currently was not needed. He returned with a big grin and told me we were moving! He had persuaded the staff to let us use that room as it meant I could have a proper bed, but obviously if it was needed for other patients then we could move back. My hero! Not quite as impressive as the suite at the hotel, but in these circumstances it was a huge improvement. We even had a small television in this room.

By that second night we all felt better. I settled down more easily in a real bed and as it was quieter and the lights were much dimmer away from the nurse's station, I felt almost like I could sleep. I drifted off but still at two-hourly intervals I was disturbed, even if only briefly. The nurse did her best to be quiet but I was alert to every noise. Dominic was miserable on and off throughout the night and little could pacify him. At 4 a.m. we agreed he was hungry so she passed him to me for a feed. She came back a few minutes later with a drink for me and she chatted to me as she changed him and settled him back in his cot. It was as if my mother was there. All that was missing was being tucked in and kissed myself! Such basics of nursing do not need great qualifications but they are so vital and appreciated. I think I actually managed to sleep until seven then.

Instead of waking up to the buzz of Dominic's christening, I woke to the sounds of the ward. Granny H arrived shortly after breakfast when he was upset again and I still had not been able to get dressed. She paced the room with him for me and he eventually fell asleep on her. I then had a blissful shower and got dressed, feeling more relaxed. Throughout the day he continued to be fretful and my mother eased the afternoon by helping me with him. Nick came at lunchtime then returned in the evening. Dominic seemed a bit brighter and the three of us watched *Robin Hood* on the tiny television. His body was under constant attack by staff with injections for him. The splint on his arm used to make me feel terrible, as I knew how uncomfortable they were.

That night was another bad one as Dominic was miserable for most of it. The nurses even tried to make us comfortable together in my bed in an attempt to settle him, but to no avail. He was still cross and bothered the next morning when two different doctors tried to take more blood samples from him. Nick came again after he had been at school for a few hours for a preparation day, but he now was not feeling too well. The tablets had affected him but not me. Both our mothers visited and my colleague Glenda again, who brought me up to date with any school news or gossip, followed later by my father and my grandparents. All these visitors definitely were appreciated and helped to keep my spirits up. As the day progressed Dominic seemed to settle down again although his voice sounded croaky. They took even more tests as his condition was proving to be a mystery and it was not meningitis. A problem with his blood platelets had shown up and they mentioned Kawasaki disease. None of us knew what this was. His bottom had become red raw due to the antibiotics and the nurses recommended we used 'Metanium', an old-fashioned but excellent cream.

After a better night Dominic seemed very hungry and could not get enough milk from me. He even began to fall asleep whilst he was still sucking – a habit he had not done since he was very tiny. When he was awake he was very quiet and lay so still. From time to time from his cot he would stare across at me through the bars with huge, deep eyes with an almost quizzical but pained expression, as though he was thinking 'Why me?' I loved to see him watching me but this used to really pull on my heartstrings. Nick had brought in the latest photographs of our trip to Corby and the filtered ones the night before he was ill. All that seemed such a long time ago, yet it was only days. I put my favourite ones up on the pin board in the room. Staff and visitors alike would comment on them and they gave me hope that we would have such times again. His cot was decorated with a few helium balloons now which he liked to watch and knock and he had been given plenty of new cuddly toys as get-well gifts. Nick came again and caused me more worry as he was ashen, weary and not at all well. He still insisted in returning for a second time later in the day. His mother had a stint with Dominic whilst I had a wander down to the hospital café for a change of scene. My mother arrived too via Chester hospital where she had just taken my grandmother to be admitted for her skin graft operation! She would go back and collect my grandfather later. Although I was tired in the hospital, I was very aware of all the running around the family were having to do in supporting each other and I appreciated it.

Some nights Dominic slept through his intravenous antibiotic – but not this one. He woke every two hours, crying loudly. Obviously I was very tired the next morning but the visitors kept me going, along with the kindness of the staff. Poor Nick was still suffering badly but a few chuckles from Dominic cheered us all up that evening. Next morning he woke in a happy mood and spent the morning kicking his legs and being fussed over by our favourite nurse, Glynis. If she was passing to go to another room she would suddenly appear, announce she had come to pinch a cuddle, make him chuckle and disappear again. I think we were all delighted to see him being so responsive. As usual the grandmothers came again plus Auntie Glynis and they too looked relieved at his progress. A huge step forward was made that evening when they took his intravenous line out and said he would now be fine taking medicine. Hurray! I could cuddle him again properly! My enthusiasm was not shared by Dominic though as I then had a very difficult evening with him.

A week after he had been admitted the doctor said he could go home. One young doctor had mainly seen him and we were glad of the continuity and confidence this provided. No real diagnosis was ever given to us except that he had indeed been a very poorly baby and it was mostly likely to have been a viral form of septicaemia. The doctor said that Dominic would be seen again at the outpatients in six weeks. When he and the nurse left the room I burst into tears – relief, exhaustion, worry? Who knows? I phoned my mother and she came for us. I packed up and the nurses gave Dominic their final cuddles, we bid our goodbyes and came home. Although I was exhausted, I knew I felt better than on the drive there and felt so grateful for all the attention we had received from everyone. We could not fault the whole staff on that ward for their care and compassion with us all. Our closest family members had also been a terrific support and I would have really struggled without them. It is the simplest of actions and gestures which are appreciated so much if you are a parent staying with a child in hospital, even if it is just someone bringing you a cup of tea.

Once at home the truth sunk in. I was now faced with the dilemma of going back to work next week. Yet Dominic was now only being breast-fed again. Both of us had not really had longer than two hours of continuous sleep for almost two weeks and were exhausted. I also simply did not want to leave him. Where to from here?

CHAPTER 10

Pressure, pressure

I felt in a daze when we both got home again and seemed to drift along. We reverted to our usual visits to family and friends in an endeavour to 'pick up the pieces' and recover from our ordeal. One good thing was that I now could fit into my jeans. I could not breathe but I could fasten them! Dominic was not sleeping well at all after having been disturbed so much by his illness. In the daytime he had periods of severe irritability and then for no apparent reason would be all smiles, usually for his grandmother. Physically his development was fine, making progress in that he could play with his toes, almost rolled from his back onto his front and could hold items midline with two hands. My GP had signed a sick note for me whilst I was in hospital with Dominic for two weeks so initially I did not need to worry about my absence. Nick said they were coping fine at school and as I would soon be back then they would manage.

When Nick went to work for the first time that September I became even more tired. He still did not look well after the side-effects of the anti-meningitis drug so I tried desperately hard for him not to be disturbed during the nights. As Dominic was waking every few hours I put him in with me in the small bed, so I did not really rest. I went to the church coffee morning on the Monday where everyone was so kind to us both and pleased to see Dominic looking well. When we came home I sobbed and sobbed due to the extreme tiredness I was feeling. Claire came at lunchtime when I was trying, without much success, to feed Dominic his lunch. I remember being very defensive about how well I was coping and tried to convince her that he would soon be eating again and sleeping and that I would be fine to go back to work in a week or two. I was jumpy and snappy in all my replies to her and flitted from extreme moods. I did not convince her and she told our mother later that although Dominic was fine, it was now me who was causing concern. 'Rubbish, I'm fine,' was my reply to that.

Next day we slept until mid-morning but as I had said I would take my grandmother to Chester hospital to have her dressings changed on her skin graft, it resulted in me panicking as we were late. We called on Sue and Ben. She admitted that she was also very worried about me. At least Dominic ate plenty of solids at teatime and he had generally had a more balanced day mood-wise. Nick began to bathe him most nights now as I suppose he could see I needed a break. We went to an NCT coffee morning and I was the centre of attention when Sue (Sophie's mother) told them about our dramatic hospital stay and I quite enjoyed telling them all about it. We then called to see Granny H. Throughout the latest hospital stay she had been a great support to us both and I was pleased in the aftermath that she and I were closer and she had no hesitation now in cuddling Dominic. As a young mother herself she had to cope with Glenys and Nick having polio. Both had been in isolation wards for weeks. Nick could only be held if she wore protective clothing and he was only a few months old then. She must have suffered terribly at that time.

Dominic's skin was a mess when we came out of hospital. It was very dry with some red itchy patches. I took him to see our GP who prescribed various ointments and bath oils. She also realised that I needed more time off work and gave me a sick note for another two weeks. She said that I was obviously very tired and still had not recovered from the trauma of Dominic's illness. I felt relieved but ended up in bed early that night with a bad headache. Nick gently suggested that I should take life a bit easier without running around here and there. He had begun to tread carefully with me as I could verbally fly off the handle at the simplest of suggestions. Next day I did my version of relaxing by cleaning the house, ironing and cooking a proper meal. I was my own worst enemy.

By mid-September, for my mother's birthday, we went for a family day out to Hawkstone Park and Follies near Whitchurch. It has pleasant walks and unusual natural and manmade areas to explore. Claire, Mum, Dad, Nick, Dominic and I all had a good day. The sun shone and because there were plenty of us to fuss Dominic he was a very contented baby. Again I tried to convince everyone that I was fine and soon would be fit for work. At times like this I probably did appear quite like my usual calm, organised self and did a reasonable job of fooling people. Nick made us have a quiet time the next day and we went to my parents for our evening meal. This became a regular event on a Sunday and it was their way of helping us. Dominic's daytime routines were slowly coming back, as regards sleeping and feeding, and he was not quite as clingy to me and did not cry or scream as much. He was still very disturbed at night, however, waking two or three times and taking a while each time to settle again. Meanwhile I continued to be very tired and had become very weepy at the least thing. Even a slight struggle opening a pot of yoghurt could reduce me to tears and any minor spillage could make me sob profusely. Everything I did was becoming increasingly hard, and such an effort. Dominic's improvements, like becoming excited when he saw his spoon and jar of food, almost passed me by.

Yet I continued to keep us both busy. If I stayed in all day Dominic seemed more fretful, which I could not handle, and as he now enjoyed going out it seemed to be the easier option. If I kept busy I also did not feel as tired. The next week passed by with shopping, going to our various coffee mornings and taking my grandparents for hospital appointments. One evening I did phone my mother in tears and ask her to have Dominic for a few hours. I needed some time away from him. He was still aggravated by his itchy skin and I went back to the GP the next day. She actually asked more about me than Dominic, which puzzled me at the time as I was fine, wasn't I?

Following on from our successful day out at Hawkstone Park I suggested that we all had another trip out. This time we went for a walk around Jumbles Country Park, near Bolton. The walk was good but all the places we had coffee, lunch and tea were problematic in one way or another and Dominic did not settle, leading to more stress. I had begun to feel that it was only me who could solve his distress. For a while this was true in hospital but now I was blind to the fact that others could soothe him too. I was still breast-feeding him regularly and usually this would comfort him, something that no one else could offer him. I felt indispensable to him and although the family tried to help me I was like a spoilt child with a new doll. He was mine and no one else was allowed to get near.

The following morning Nick kept Dominic with him whilst he did his chores and left me to rest and sleep. Instead I read the newspaper which contained an article about postnatal depression. My belief that I was 'not the type' to have such a thing and that my problems were purely due to tiredness began to dispel. As I read the symptoms of mood swings, tiredness, irritability, weepiness, I recognised myself. They suggested antidepressant tablets as a cure but I immediately dismissed that idea as I did not need drugs; I just needed a rest which was also a suggestion. I felt optimistic that maybe after a few good nights of sleep everything would be all right again. At my parents for a meal that evening, Dominic ate plenty of food and even had more porridge when we came home. I felt convinced that we would all be fine and had a couple of good days.

Ray, the vicar, had encouraged Nick and I to attend a series of weekly discussion groups questioning the Christian faith, called Alpha classes. As both of us were not sure about our true beliefs, it seemed a good idea and we hoped to make some new friends. It also meant that we did something as a couple and my parents would babysit for us for a couple of hours. I felt very guilty going to the classes initially as I had always been brought up to believe that if you were not fit for school or work then you should not be out socialising. Everyone else said I needed to get out to help me feel better, so we went. It was good to break away from everything at home but really it was not an ideal time for me to join in religious debates. I was so confused about everything in my own life at that stage, so having to contribute to group discussions added even more pressures. It was refreshing though to hear some points of view from firm believers in the Christian faith. I felt envious of the calmness and peace that they appeared to have about life. I had now begun to get worried about mundane aspects, such as what to make for a meal, yet these people appeared to float through life. I wanted to feel such contentment and spiritually rich.

I continued with our outings and I took Dominic to his first Mums and Tots swimming session. I really enjoyed it with him. I still had great maternal pleasure in holding him, especially when he was so vulnerable in the water and he clung to me for security. I loved his smell, especially his hair. I loved to watch his movements. I was fascinated by his increasing social awareness which drove me forward to take him to more places. Consequently I was not content with the one outing and we then had lunch with Sue and Sophie, went to a church group and called at my grandparents before coming home. I made Nick and I a proper meal and spent ages liquidising some of it for Dominic. He spat it out. I got upset. Nick reprimanded me for doing too much again. I said I had to keep busy as I would not survive at work if I spent my time now lazing around. Luckily Nick took over Dominic for the rest of the evening whilst he made me 'just sit'.

This was followed by another really disturbed night and I moped around all morning in my dressing gown, bemoaning my current situation. My mother phoned to see how I was and suggested that as my father was not working, why not let him look after Dominic for a few hours? I did so and spent a few hours making myself look presentable for Ben's second birthday party that afternoon. I collected Dominic, changed him into his smart wedding outfit and off we went. Sue was due to go into hospital the next day to have a Caesarean. She was very weary too and in comparison I felt slim and awake! In reality, in my worst spells I felt just as exhausted as a heavily pregnant mother-to-be. Our health visitor came out to see us again. She wrote in Dominic's record book that I needed more sleep and was not on top of things at present. I felt offended. Of course I was!

Back at the GP's the next day, I had more creams for Dominic's 'sandpaper' skin and once again she spent a while talking to me. She sighed, put her pen down and looked at me. She explained that she felt now that my moods and feelings were not just due to the trauma and stress of Dominic's illness but that I was indeed suffering from postnatal depression. This was usually caused by hormonal and medical changes although, in my case, the other stresses I had been under may have made it worse. When I told her that I had read an article about it and had recognised some of my symptoms too, so agreed with her, I almost felt she was relieved. She suggested that I tried some tablets which would help me to relax and sleep, when I could, but also that they may help me feel more on top of things. She continued to say that they were not an instant cure and that they would take a few weeks to take effect, but in her opinion they were worth me trying. I told her that I felt antidepressant drugs were for people 'who could not cope' and that once I started on them then I would be addicted for life – common assumptions by many people. She disagreed on both aspects and stressed that I had an illness that would be helped by medication, just like any other complaint. I still felt though that it was purely because I was inadequate but I was willing to try them. She signed me off for a further four weeks. Part of me felt relief that I had longer off but equally I felt terribly guilty for the problems I knew it would cause at school as they were having trouble finding a suitable supply teacher. I phoned them hesitantly but the head teacher told me not to worry but to get well soon. We then went to visit Cathy as we had decided that maybe Dominic should start spending some time with her.

In a way I suppose I was quite relieved to be told that I had an identifiable illness because it gave me something to hang a label onto. I have always loved 'projects' ever since junior school days. I love researching and planning, just as I did before Dominic was born. When postnatal depression (PND) was diagnosed, I looked it up in every medical book we had and homed in on any relevant articles in magazines. Nick and I were especially alert to any form of help and consequently I discovered and wrote to the Association for Post Natal Illness [see contact details in the Appendix]. Their newsletter was useful with short articles on past and present sufferers and fundraising. One of the services they offer is a telephone link with a former sufferer as a means of support. I did get a number and name but I can not remember if I got in touch. They continue to send me newsletters and raffle tickets so I am well aware that there are still many people suffering from this condition, and it is one reason why I am writing all of this. It was through one of their articles that I read about a lady who was researching the area. Later on she came to interview me about my experiences as part of her studies. They also sent a useful booklet about PND, notes for the carer and a leaflet on puerperal psychosis, the most severe form of the illness. I read it and dismissed it as almost ridiculous. How on earth anyone would want to harm themselves and their baby was beyond me. However, all the leaflets were of help and we let our families and close friends look at them. We even sent them into school for the head to look at.

I found a copy of a letter which I wrote to my college friends, Margaret and Richard, around this time. It shows how I was feeling and that at least I was prepared to tell my friends – on paper.

> When Dominic was discharged from hospital and we came home it was like him being newborn, as there were no rules again. The diagnosis was that he'd had a viral septicaemia which left much longer would have gone to his spine, then brain ... luckily we got him there in time.
>
> The trauma for us has been awful. Nick and I had to take an anti-meningitis drug which made him poorly too and he missed the start of term. He is now back at work but I am not. Initially I was, and still am, exhausted as Dominic still does not sleep for

more than three hours at a time and, instead of the happy, contented baby he was, is much more demanding and whingy. He is improving but unfortunately I appear to be showing classic postnatal depression symptoms! School will just have to wait as at the moment thinking out what I should cook for dinner is causing me great anxiety and panic attacks, so I'd not be much use in a classroom. Since February I have had a total of 28 nights in hospital which is now telling on me. Prior to these last few weeks I admit I had no sympathy with PND sufferers, but I have now!

I hope that as Dominic continues to improve, I will to. We just feel so upset that all was okay until he was so poorly. I wouldn't wish that experience on anyone. I am now trying to find a balance between resting and yet not staying in all that much. If I'm on my own I want company and yet when I'm in company I want to be by myself!

Enough wallowing ...

My friend Sue, who you met at our wedding, is due in hospital for a section on Thursday as the baby is breach. That is Ben's 2nd birthday so he is having his party a day earlier this year – I've been asked to help with the jelly, etc. I should cope with that! She will then have the baby on Friday because she said she didn't want them to share the same birthday. I don't think I could manage two yet!

I had better finish as there is a screaming baby lying on the floor next to me!'

By the time Dominic was five months old he weighed 18 lbs 1 oz and was 67.5 cm long. He had no regular sleep or feeding patterns due to his illness but had recently begun a range of pureed foods in addition to breast milk. His favourite tastes were pears, carrots, porridge, beans and bacon (tinned), and fromage frais with fruit. He had developed dry and rough patches on his skin but his health was reasonable in general. He could lift his head up, watch his hands, roll onto his side then to his front and loved to play with his toes. He had longer hair and smiled a lot more at people and things. He had developed a range of happy sounds and would 'talk' to us frequently.

He did not have a 'typical' day at this stage. Neither did I.

CHAPTER 11

Losing it!

Dominic's sixth month began on a few positive notes. He stayed with Cathy for a couple of hours successfully whilst I went to the dentist and shopped. We went to a coffee morning with Sue C and Sophie, then after lunch he had his first swing in the playground at Walton Gardens. That evening, Nick and I went to buy a second cot for Dominic to have at my parents' house. He was now not safe to leave just in his pram and we all intended that in due course he would stay the night occasionally with them to give us a rest. Next day was a lucky one as we won £10 on the lottery and received a letter from a shop to say Dominic had won the prize draw for a go-kart. At an NCT sale we went to at Tarporley, I found a beautiful designer christening outfit for Dominic at a bargain price. He was now too big for the original one and we had arranged another date. Due to our current high involvement with the church, Ray had agreed to christen him during one of the usual Sunday morning communion services instead. I was pleased as not only did it mean we could share the experience with some of our new friends, but we could now also book a lunch out afterwards. Great – things were looking up again. Dominic had improved his eating and was learning new skills every day. He had discovered his fingernails and loved to scratch surfaces, including his head, leaving marks – the health visitor noted them. I remember thinking that I was a suspect as I now was a drug addict and failing mother!

I carried on that week with our timetable of visits and shopping but a step forward was made by Nick leaving Dominic with Cathy on Thursday and Friday mornings on his way to work. She had two boys who were five and three years old and they treated Dominic like an adopted little brother. I had been in the same geography 'A' level class during my sixth form days as her husband – what a small world. I was quite happy leaving him there and felt that it was good to have some time apart so it would not be such a wrench when I did go back to work full time. This also meant that I had two mornings a week to myself and everyone stressed to me that I was to rest and not be running around trying to catch up on tasks. For a few weeks I did heed advice and especially liked reading the local newspapers in bed with my breakfast as soon as Nick and Dominic left. After about half an hour I would slide under the covers and doze off again. Why do postmen, window cleaners, meter readers and double-glazing sales people choose such mornings to ring the doorbell? I must have developed a reputation as a very rude, lazy person through my dealings with them and I definitely pitied night-shift workers. I still had to give Dominic up to three feeds during the night and I had begun to lose any body clock system I once had.

At the start of the next week I admitted to myself that I was too tired to go to the church hall so we stayed in and had a lazy morning. I had got dressed just before lunchtime when my head teacher called to see how I was getting along. Luckily Dominic was asleep throughout her visit and after a few minutes of talking to her I found myself in 'school mode' and chatted enthusiastically about plans for my class. I reassured her that I did want to come back and that I was becoming a bit tired of talking to people about brands of nappies and baby foods. A fog seemed to lift and I got caught up in my own wave of excitement that had dawned on me – yes, there was still Elaine Hanzak, the efficient teacher, lurking there. We reminisced about this time last year when I had been giving countywide lectures on teaching 16–19 year-old pupils in special schools and both spoke of our hopes that I would soon be back to it. I was not bluffing during our conversation as I honestly felt that I wanted to go back to being a complete person again and to prove I could do it all. I was even still quite high about it when Nick came in from work that afternoon. I do not think he was convinced.

When I awoke next day I was low again. I took Dominic swimming but did not enjoy it. We came home and I sat and cried until I felt I had no tears left. What on earth had I been thinking yesterday? I could not cope with my child and myself at the moment, so how on earth could I handle teaching a class too? I was failing as a person, a mother and as a wife. To fail too as a teacher would just be too much. Somehow, after this outburst, I cheered up and went to visit Sue and her new baby girl, Katie.

Lucky Sue – she had one of each now. Both she and the lovely tiny baby were well and I was pleased to see them. I still felt very raw about my birth experience and wanted to cry again as Sue told me about her time in hospital. I often wanted to do an 'action replay' now of the last few months, but that was impossible. She asked how I was. 'Fine' was my reply. I know she did not believe me. After our evening meal both Nick and I were pleased when Dominic watched us open and close our hands and he copied us! He was now starting to achieve things that some of the children we taught could not do and every tiny stage impressed and amazed us. That week I noticed that Nick too had begun to be cross about mundane matters more than usual, such as waiting too long for the car to have its MOT. He must have been finding our lifestyle very trying and yet I was powerless to help or even notice. Little by little I was distancing myself from the people I was closest to. I am normally an affectionate and demonstrative person but I had begun to recoil from hugs given to offer me support. I did not need them, I told myself.

Instead of relaxing on my next mornings off, I arranged to see a support worker who was going to be running a group for up to six local mothers who were currently diagnosed as suffering from PND. It would run for a few weeks and we would cover a whole range of topics to 'help us cope with everything more successfully'. Although I was willing to go and try anything which may help me, her comment about such sufferers 'not being able to cope' further convinced me that I was a failure. Consequently the next morning I went to a Tupperware party without Dominic, instead of resting. I had to prove to the world that I was managing. Later that day Dominic and I went to my antenatal class reunion. All the other four babies were now virtually sleeping through every night and none of the others were still breast-feeding as much as I was. On the group photograph we set up with the camera on timer, Dominic is the only screaming baby and I look very pale and gaunt. I always liked meeting this group and all the other mums were genuinely sympathetic. I just felt stupid having all these problems.

The end of the summer had arrived, and that weekend I wrapped Dominic up so he could sit outside whilst his Dad washed, dismantled and put away the garden furniture. We had an autumnal walk around Norton Priory, a local tourist attraction. Seeing the leaves turning to rich reds and bright yellows reminded me of all the enthusiasm I had felt for life at the start of summer with our new baby. Now I felt so weary, numb to many pleasures and as if I had lost the real 'me' somewhere during the last few months.

Although I was rarely completely alone I felt very lonely inside. At junior school I was always last to be picked on the skittle-ball team and used to dread that awful feeling of rejection. I would stare at the two confident captains with pleading eyes. They would avoid them and all the physically skilled classmates would gradually leave my side to join the team. I was the useless one that nobody wanted. Disappointed. Unwanted. Rejected. That was how I now felt about myself again.

I drifted through the next week keeping Dominic and myself busy. I still wanted to help out with my grandparents as it was something I could do well, and even if it tired me, it gave me confidence. Nick and my mother always said it was too much for me but I ignored their advice – what did they know? I knew I was perfectly fine. Some nights Dominic only woke once but I kept waking up and waiting for him to cry. I even used to get up and go and check on him in his room. Sometimes I would sit in the comfy armchair in there until he did actually disturb. With Nick shut away in the back bedroom he was oblivious to my new night-time wandering. He continued to stir if Dominic cried but not anything else. If I could not sleep I might read a magazine for hours. It always seemed to be that just as I did settle then someone or something woke me and I would feel lousy.

I attended my first PND support group. There were six of us with two group leaders. One of my new friends from one of the coffee mornings was also there! We both laughed when we saw one another as neither of us had mentioned we were going, but now it meant we could actually talk to each other with more honesty and even do 'homework' together. The other ladies were of mixed ages, backgrounds and circumstances. We were all so very different but with postnatal illness affecting us all in some way. I had been trying to convince myself that I was ill and not just failing, but the first session aimed to make us all realise that there is no such thing as a perfect mother and to accept 'good enough'. In my current state of mind, this confused me. If the cause is chemical and hormone imbalance then what had our aspirations of perfection got to do with it? I asked them to clarify this for me but neither leader did to my satisfaction and they moved on to something else. We discussed a variety of issues and examples of the symptoms of our condition. Someone repeated a case they had heard about a lady who felt she was engulfed at times in extreme waves of wanting to hurt herself. Apparently her GP had told her that there were other ways to get attention than this and as she would not take the medication he had prescribed, then there was little more he could do! We were all horrified by this story but some of us identified with the reluctance of this lady to take antidepressants, for example knowing about people who had taken them and become addicted. At that point our allotted time was up and we were told that the session was over until next week. Although most of the group left feeling more positive, my reaction was that I felt ruffled and worse than when I had gone in, due to my interpretation of the issues. I knew I did like everything to be perfect but I did not feel it was fair to imply that it was the cause of all this. Oh no! I had brought it all on my family and myself. I now had guilt to contend with too.

Seeing Sue, Ben and baby Katie lifted my spirits later and Sue reassured me that the sessions would probably get better. By the time Nick came home I was more positive and tried to focus on telling him about the other sufferers. In a way it was a comfort to know we were not alone – more new parents were struggling too. One lady had been great after her first two babies but was suffering badly after the arrival of her third even though financially they were better off and knew what to expect of a baby. We came to the conclusion that we had just been unlucky.

I did try now to leave Dominic with others more often. His two mornings with Cathy were going well. He went to my parents quite regularly and we used to leave him with Nick's mother sometimes whilst he and I went shopping. My mother-in-law lived about 25 minutes drive away from us and often commented that she would have helped more if we were closer. I was becoming more relaxed about being apart and at times was very pleased to be away from his demands. Yet this too added to my guilt. Dominic had begun to make progress in sitting up so we lowered his cot down one level and at the same time bagged up more of his outgrown clothes for the loft. The thought of a 'next time' irritated and annoyed me. As I folded each item they brought back a whole range of emotions – happy summer walks, sorrowful hospital stays, exhausted nights. I buried my face in a misnamed 'sleep suit' and sobbed to Nick, asking him 'Why is it all so hard? Why does he not sleep? Why is life so difficult? Why do I feel so useless?'

He did his best to console me but I guess he was at a loss for the answers too. My newborn baby was no more, like my dreams for a blissful family life. In reality, every day was an uphill struggle and I never got to the top of the mountain I was attempting to climb. I was a hamster in a wheel, running and running but going nowhere.

I did like going to my parents for our Sunday dinner as they always made a fuss over Dominic, we had a good meal and I often found a task I could do. That particular day, talking about our loft trip at home and putting his clothes away, reminded us of the treasure trove in my parents' loft, especially as we remembered that there were toys from our childhood days. As soon as we had eaten I climbed up there and lost myself in sorting, searching, rummaging and finding many of Claire's toddler toys. Such tasks were very therapeutic as I was able to concentrate and forget my self-pity and exhaustion. The adrenaline flowed and put me on a high for a while in spite of family cries that I 'was doing too much'. They just did not realise that I had to find something I was good at, to prove that I was still a useful human being. Then we went back home and I was woken three times in the night.

Next day we went to a coffee morning. It was cancelled so I came back and vacuumed and tidied the house, neither of which really needed doing but I had to be busy. Nick would be pleased, I told myself, but obviously he would rather I had relaxed and watched television. More visiting, more shopping, more screaming from Dominic. Another disturbed night. I must keep busy though. Jeannie and Oliver came to see us. We went to Mums and Tots. We visited my grandparents. I just could not stop. I had to keep busy to tell Nick interesting things. If I stayed in I would become a bore. Men don't like bores. We were not passionate these days. He must have gone off me. Keep busy and he will fancy me again. (Poor man was exhausted too.) Somehow this is how my mind began to work – short, sharp reasoning that was gradually becoming illogical.

At the next support group we had to complete a task about who was important to us in our lives and who had the most influence. We had to choose a clothes button which we felt represented ourself, then choose and position other family members around us on a sheet of card. I had great trouble in seeing the difference in identifying Dominic as a huge, shining, bright and loud button in contrast to myself as a tatty, chipped and faded, pale shirt button! Normally I would have enjoyed the symbolism of this activity. At that session one of the group told us about a sufferer she had heard about who had locked herself in her bathroom and torn at her forearms with her razor. Upon discovering this scene her mother had then taken her to the doctor's who had asked why she had done it. She explained she did not know why, other than this wave of self-harming that inexplicably came over her. He apparently tutted and said that if she must do such things then she should do it properly and cut up the arm instead of across as it was more effective for blood loss. We were all stunned and appalled by this story but appreciative of the support we were all receiving. My sympathy went out to another member of the group who was obviously having a bad day. I really wanted to help her but due to my own vulnerable state, I could not. My feelings towards the group leaders were extreme, due to my state of health, as they apparently just let her walk out whilst they chatted about their social plans. I felt shocked and disgusted that they could let her go. Maybe I saw myself in her, and it was really me shouting inside 'Somebody help'. However, my faith and hope in that group left with that lady as she walked out through the door. I know that the other group members felt that it helped them and I still continued to attend each week even though it did not feel right for me. I withdrew further into myself, refusing to add much to the discussions. I was just a tiny, tarnished button after all.

From this I catapulted myself into lunch out at a pub with Sue C and Sophie when I had collected Dominic. After a visit to the baby clinic I later walked to school to meet Nick and hand in yet another sick note. I felt extremely uncomfortable as everyone fussed over Dominic and commented on how well I looked. See! I knew it! They think I'm a big skiver. I've always been a wimp and now they all know it's true. I looked well, so I must be. I am imagining all my fears and failures. Yes, I will be back very soon, of course I will. I am much better. Dominic gave Nick a huge smile of recognition when he saw him and put his arms out to go to him. The staff gushed and teased that the baby must like him after all. I wanted to disappear under the carpet and hide as the big fraud I obviously was. I still felt guilty about being out and about when I was not fit for work and this visit had made it all worse.

Reassured later by Nick, he encouraged me to carry on with the following day I had arranged. I had won a beauty makeover at a salon in Warrington. My parents were to have Dominic all day for me and indeed I did relax as best as I could. I had always wanted a very special and beautiful photograph of me with my baby, like the best ones you see in a photographer's window, with a soft filter, misty eyes and a bare child against bare shoulders. Nick said he could do this for us so that early evening we tried a whole variety of poses, none of which were very good! Yet another failure. Dominic looked tired and bored and he was covered in little scratches he had given himself. In spite of my beauty treatment I look washed out and my hair is too heavy at the sides. Undeterred, Granny H came to babysit for us that night whilst we went out for a meal together for the first time in ages. I was quiet and not much company. He did not find me attractive any more so what was the point of making an effort? I had failed with my first marriage so I was not likely to make a success of my second, was I?

Without Dominic's diary I would have now found it almost impossible to remember him as he reached six months old as I was becoming more aloof and detached from him as I became more insular. My highs were few and far between; a balanced, sensible outlook rare; being low was now most common. However, as I look back at Dominic's photographs at that time, he had grown into a cute baby with an endearing smile which attracted attention wherever we went. He now weighed 18 lbs, 8 oz and was 70 cm long. He slept in his nursery between 8 p.m. and 8 a.m., with up to four wakes a night, and had a morning and afternoon nap. His meals were now a savoury and sweet puree or tinned baby fruit followed by water from a cup with a soft spout. He still had breast-feeds too. Apart from his skin complaint his health had been good and the health visitor always commented how alert and bright he appeared. He could roll from his front to back now, reached and twisted his body to touch and scratch things and could flick his spinning rattle. His hair was beginning to regrow on top and his eyes were turning more green/brown, like mine. His repertoire of sounds had increased to blowing raspberries, gurgling, 'uuh-uuh' and 'arh'. He loved being played with, being dangled in his door bouncer, rolling over and holding things. His favourite outings were shopping, swimming and car journeys in general.

Who was this child that everyone fussed over? Was he anything to do with me? I did not know anymore.

CHAPTER 12

Downhill

As British summer time ended that year both Nick and Dominic developed a cold, making them quite grumpy. One statement of advice in the Mothercare diary that week was regarding common illnesses. It read 'if your baby is ill, you will have to drop everything else and dedicate yourself to looking after him'. We were well experienced in this! All three of us went to communion that Sunday morning where we worked hard to keep Dominic from disturbing the congregation. I felt we should go as he was soon to be christened.

Our health visitor came out to see us. Nick was on half-term holiday and I think she wanted to check how we all were managing. We stressed that it was Dominic's erratic sleeping pattern which was still our main cause for concern, making us all tired, especially me. She was sympathetic and offered some advice. She reminded me of how I must have appeared to parents when I taught nursery children – young, single, no children, well meaning and knowledgeable from reading books and writing essays – but it was very hard to try to make her really understand the pressure we were all under. She was always pleasant and did her best to help us. Just her presence and willingness to listen were often a tonic. At times I know I did put on a false impression to her and tried to hide my feelings of inadequacy by chatting incessantly about all the places we had been. On that particular visit she complimented me on the progress I had made with Dominic's eating. Thus, inspired, I spent a while making him a proper, homemade puree full of goodness for his tea. He spat it out at me. I could not even cook these days, it seemed. In my first marriage we had been in the 'dinner party' mode socially and I used to be able to make a five course meal to a high standard. Now I could not even cook and mash carrots satisfactorily.

Nick's second morning off was spent in a chaotic waiting room at the general hospital for an outpatient's appointment for Dominic as a follow-up to his illness. The three of us waited for almost two hours – not easy with a six-month-old baby in a tiny room full of other fractious children and parents. There was never any indication as to how long we had to wait. If we had been told we could have at least gone for a stroll and a drink. When you wait at Accident and Emergency departments you know you have to be dealt with in order of severity and it is easier to cope with, as you understand the reason. Yet why you should have to wait two hours for an outpatient appointment is a mystery. When we were eventually seen it was by a doctor who had never met any of us before. He had to read through Dominic's records and listen to us before he could pass any comment. We told him about his disturbed sleep pattern and rough skin. He noted his runny nose and mentioned that he may have infant colic but otherwise he seemed fine. He reassured us that all these problems would settle down in time and that we should not worry. We both left feeling rather ruffled and irritable after the whole morning's experiences. To console ourselves we had our first family trip to McDonalds for lunch! After the Lake District experience we were both reluctant to dine out with him at formal restaurants.

The rest of the half-term week passed with jobs around the house and at my parents, shopping and trying to recover from colds. Dominic was doing well, now rolling confidently from his back to front then back again. He had started to push up on his hands whilst on his front and move his legs. He shook rattles by bending his wrist as opposed to his whole arm and made a sound when you patted his lips. He also did this to himself and would happily lay in his pram 'blubbing' his lips. I was still desperate to know how to get him to sleep better but everywhere I turned for help, either by reading or being told, the advice contradicted itself. Some recommended a rigid routine, others said flexibility was the answer. Some said let him sleep with you, others dismissed this as ridiculous and once you started this there would be no end to it. Friends and relatives also tried to give me advice. I did try it all but still nothing seemed to work. The latest problem was that his cold had left him with a nasty cough, which disturbed us even more.

Yet again I was back at our surgery. This time Dominic was given anti-biotics and an inhaler for bronchiolitis. He did actually sleep a little better, just waking at 4 a.m. and 5.30 a.m. most mornings. I was so used to the small hours now that I was awake regardless. I just could not seem to sleep properly any more, even when I had the chance. By the middle of that week we decided that as I could not settle across the landing from him and that Nick was being just as disturbed and not coping, we should make alternative plans. I desperately needed Nick to be functioning properly. If he was tired and bad tempered that made me worse, so we had to do what we felt best, regardless of all the contradictory advice. Consequently we decided to move Dominic's cot into our bedroom and let Nick retreat back into the small bedroom. The theory was that I could sleep better, and if necessary put him in with me in the big bed. Sleep was more important than ethics at this stage!

That weekend Nick and I went out together for a meal at the Lord Dares-bury hotel. This was more successful than our last evening out, but as neither of us were particularly lively we just ate and came home to sleep in separate rooms. I still knew I had lost my spark along the way and even a simple pleasure like this was a huge effort. At least we had learnt not to be quite as busy at weekends and only tried to do a sensible level of shopping, visiting and outings. Sunday dinner at my parents was well established now and continued to be a success. Dominic loved his door bouncer on loan from Sophie and once in it would spend ages just bobbing around. It proved invaluable at mealtimes as he could watch us all whilst we ate and he would dine after us. We took it to my parents' too.

The following morning Nick was poorly so Dominic and I kept out of the house to let him rest. Sue C had hurt her foot and needed an X-ray and, as we were free, we took her and spent more time in a waiting room. The next day Dominic had a temperature so I took him to the doctor's. He tried to imply that I was getting overcautious now about every little complaint that Dominic presented. He reassured me that although he understood how his hospital stay had alarmed us all, now we must accept that just like any infant Dominic would pick up germs that just needed time and a little paracetamol to solve them. I came away feeling like a fussing mother. By early evening he was violently sick several times and just drooped across my lap for hours. He was the same the next day and did not keep down the paracetamol I gave him. I refused to go back to the doctor's because obviously I was making it all out to be worse than it was. Nick went instead and got antibiotics for a throat infection. Next morning Dominic was diagnosed with the same problem and also needed antibiotics. By now at least at the surgery we did not need to spell out our unusual surname (as we regularly have to) as they knew us well!

By the weekend Dominic was much better and we carried on with our plans. My parents had discovered discounted leisure breaks at hotels and often would go away for a treat. A few years earlier, when Claire had been working in Reading, we had met up with her for a weekend at the Merryhill Copthorne Hotel at Dudley in the Midlands. It had a leisure club and was next to the Merryhill shopping centre. My mother suggested we should go there again and we thought Dominic would like the Christmas decorations. Granny H had bought him the next stage car seat as an early Christmas present and we christened it on this outing. He was quite cosy in it. On this stay it was just my mother, Claire, Dominic and I sharing two rooms. The plan was that we could put Dominic to sleep in one room whilst we watched television and I took our baby monitor so we could listen if there was a problem. However, the rooms were too far apart for it to work!

The first night he woke frequently. Claire was sharing with us and she could not believe how many times he woke up. Once again I chatted incessantly about how it was not a problem; of course I handled it okay and in a few weeks I would probably be off the tablets. I did not need them anyway, I tried to convince her. We spent the Saturday mooching around the shops, each taking it in turns to push or carry Dominic around. My mother decided to have her hair done whilst we were there. To our great amusement when we all went for a swim in the hotel pool on our return, a boy jumped in by her, soaking her freshly blow-dried hair! It was a real tonic to feel myself really laugh – it was a rare occurrence these days. We bought a selection of goodies for a bedroom picnic back at the hotel and had a relaxed evening, drinking and eating. Dominic settled well to sleep in with his grandmother but in the early hours woke up, and after a struggle she had to bring him to me for a feed. I put him in with me for a little while and he was sick all over both of us plus the bedding. At 3 a.m. we had to call housekeeping for more linen. It certainly gave Claire an insight into our night times! On the way home he slept blissfully in his comfortable new car seat. It had been a pleasant change of scene and no more tiring than being at home. At least Nick had been able to recover on his own.

He went back to work on the Monday but Dominic and I had been up all night due to him coughing and having wind. I had no energy to go out so we both stayed in without getting dressed until late in the afternoon. I kept crying, so did Dominic. He hardly ate all day and was very bad tempered. I managed to cheer up when Nick came home but we then had a difficult evening and very restless night again. I was beginning to despair. Next morning I chatted to both Sues for moral support. They both said I should go back to the doctor's with him. I was reluctant to do so but made an appointment. The thought of driving the car seemed too much so I phoned my father, in tears, and he immediately came over. After another inconclusive doctor visit my father insisted we all went to their house. He made me go to bed and kept Dominic amused and happy for hours. Why couldn't I do that? All he did for me was scream (or so it seemed). When my mother came in from work she told me that I needed a new outfit for his christening and suggested we went to look for one. I felt fat and misshapen but in the end we found a jade jacket, checked skirt and bright blue jumper which were ideal. At least the bright colours did not make me feel frumpy and it was comfortable. Retail therapy can help sometimes.

After a relatively good night when I was up only three times, I still did not feel like going out. My father called with my grandparents and again they amused Dominic whilst I pottered around. Nick had told me to wait for him and then we all went grocery shopping together for a change. I had been doing this myself as I had the time, I insisted, but Nick was realising that even this was now becoming a strain. Naturally he wanted to help as much as he could, but I was obstinate and awkward when help was offered as I took it as another indication of my failure. We were all in a 'no-win' situation. I was given yet another sick note and foolishly took it into school myself and tortured myself with all the negative emotions I had experienced on the previous visit. Every time someone commented that I looked well I wanted to smack them and scream 'But I'm not!' Instead I smiled pathetically and replied, 'Yes, not too bad.' The violent reaction I had quite surprised me as I had never been that way inclined before.

With Dominic's christening approaching I went to have my hair done. I did not want it cut short but wanted to persevere with the length so I could try another perm in a few months. It left me with a strange in-between style that did not really flatter me. Even Richard commented that I was quiet. Cathy had suggested that she keep Dominic for longer so I could have lunch out by myself. I reluctantly agreed but felt very guilty as I poured myself a cup of tea. I should be working, not a 'lady who lunches'. Months earlier I had booked for Nick and I to see the stage musical *Blood Brothers*, another of my favourites. Tonight was the night and it added further to my guilt about socialising whilst not at work. For the first time ever I began to feel really scared as we walked into the circle at the theatre. My heart pounded and a wave of fright came over me as if someone had announced that there was a bomb in the building. I grabbed Nick and told him. He reassured me that I would be fine when the play started, but the close proximity of the people around me also was scaring me. I felt trapped. I could not breathe. People next to me, behind me, in front of me, below me, everywhere. People. People. High ceiling. Big stage. Noisy, so noisy.

Luckily when the curtain rose my panic feelings subsided and I lost myself in the production. The story is about twins who are separated at birth but whose paths cross regularly as they grow up. In the finale as both lay dead and their mother sings 'tell me it's not true, say it's just a story', tears rolled like peas down my cheeks. That's how I felt about my life at the moment. I had tried so hard to make everything acceptable, not perfect but good enough, yet I was getting nowhere. What else could I do? I had tried the tablets, the support group, tried to rest but it was all hopeless, hopeless. I was hopeless. I did not utter a sound the whole journey home.

Next day we had to sort out the house for the christening and both Nick and I buzzed as we cleaned. Claire had come home for the weekend and she helped to keep Dominic happy. We had bought a dummy to try him with. A few days after he was born a nurse had suggested one but he had just spat it out. Further down the line we thought it was worth another try – no chance! Nick gave him a bath as usual and as he was drying him Dominic decided to relieve himself, soaking the bathroom floor and his father!

At last his christening day dawned. It was terrible weather – hailstones, rain, wind and very cold. Our original plan of walking leisurely up to church had to be abandoned and we went in cars. Before the service Roy came and we had a photo session of baby, father and godfather. I felt quite smart in my new outfit and appreciated my mother's encouragement in getting me to find something new. I was pleased to put Dominic in his bargain outfit, which was a bit small now but acceptable. Whilst I was pregnant my mother had spent hours knitting an exquisite, delicate shawl.

I decided I wanted to use it first for his christening. I know she wanted me to use it more but equally I wanted him to have something really special for this day. His white suit was complimented by a little white hat and he looked cute. I just hoped he would be good.

When we arrived at the church the rain had stopped temporarily and we took some more photographs at the door. Little did we know then that I would be back at that very spot in due course. The congregation made us very welcome and many were now familiar faces. It was much better to feel part of the community in this way as opposed to the Sunday afternoon en-mass christening. Ray was lovely and explained about how poorly Dominic had been, making today even more special, and mentioned him throughout the service and sermon. Our son was very well behaved throughout and I would have been very proud of him except I felt numb during the whole occasion. Somehow I felt I was not there. I was just a bystander yet I knew these people well. Claire looked gorgeous in a full-length black velvet coat and was admired by many people. Roy looked quite emotional during the service, making me feel pleased that Nick had asked him to be Dominic's godfather. Sue complained that she felt huge after having Katie but nonetheless I was glad she was there too – she was a good friend to me.

We had plenty of photographs taken after the service. I look pale and strained. Nick looks tired. Dominic looks amazed and bewildered. Soon we were back home and had coffee with our family and friends. I took Dominic upstairs to change him. As he lay in his cot looking beautiful in his white outfit, surrounded by his immaculate white bedding and bright toys, I did feel quite overwhelmed by him and the occasion. I desperately wanted to feel so happy. I knew I should but why did I feel so distant from this beautiful baby? I knew that in my album of me as a child there was a picture of me wearing white and surrounded by white. I wanted to capture my son looking like me – maybe then I would feel he was really mine. There was no time though because people needed coffee and I had to serve it. No one else could do it. It was my house. My cups. My kettle. I had to do it. They all knew I was useless so I had to show I was not. Down I went – oh, someone's done it already. Huh – they all are scheming against me. I know it. It's a plot against me and I'm losing.

The arrival of my other friend Sue C from church knocked me back into some sense as I introduced her. Meanwhile the weather worsened and we ran to cars and drove through blizzard-like conditions to the hotel. Even the weather was against me. The meal for our family and friends was good but I could not relax as usual and fussed over Dominic. He was very happy being passed around his nearest and dearest but I faffed and clucked that he needed this, he needed that. In retrospect I was a nuisance! Nick made a brief speech, thanking people for coming and for the presents. He thanked me for having produced such a wonderful son, even if he did not sleep!

Lies, lies, I thought to myself. The grandparents obviously enjoyed the day and we have some good photographs of them with their grandson.

Back at home Dominic was very pleasant, with smiles and chuckles for everyone. I could not fully join in the merriment as I was already thinking of the night hours to come. Where would all these happy faces be then, I thought, as I pictured myself pacing the floor with him, trying to keep him quiet. We had tried the 'leave him crying' school of thought – it just made him and us worse. When I changed him later I did actually get the 'white' photographs of him and he does look like I did as a baby. I was demanding too. We posed too by all his lovely presents, ranging from a bible to Peter Rabbit crockery to a Liverpool football kit (from Roy, one of their biggest fans)! When our guests had gone I called to see a neighbour who had asked to see him in his outfit. On reflection the day had gone well. It was just me who these days found fault with everything and actually enjoying myself was virtually impossible as silly thoughts got in the way.

After all the excitement of the christening Dominic had me awake most of the night – see, I had anticipated and, yes, I was right, where were all those happy faces now? I took the films to be developed next day and just shopped locally. Nick was still not encouraging me to go further afield and I had begun to resist going very far. Someone had suggested that a heavy cereal at night might make Dominic sleep for longer. He did not always wake for food but I decided to give him Weetabix for supper. Only two wake-ups that night! Feeling slightly better next morning, we collected the photographs and I spent the day taking them around to show the family.

Dominic's seventh month came to a close with him now a baptised member of the Christian family. His natural family were exhausted but he was thriving. He weighed just under 19 lbs and was 70 cm long. His sleeping pattern was terrible, some nights waking up to six times. He ate well and enjoyed his food, now often dining in his highchair. He had seen a number of doctors for bronchiolitis, a sore throat and being 'off colour'. His favourite activity was jumping in his door bouncer and he liked holding and looking at objects.

Our social timetable had been drastically curtailed as I could not be bothered to make the effort to go. It meant I would have to talk to people who did not want to listen to me as I was so boring. It was better to stay in wearing my dressing gown. This whinging baby did not care, so why should I?

CHAPTER 13

The final descent

All the pressure on Nick was taking its toll and he was too ill to go to work again for a few days. Apart from all the disturbed nights and not knowing what to do to help me, he was under intense stress at work. Staff constantly asked him how I was throughout the day – just as he concentrated on something someone else would ask. They felt they should enquire and genuinely did want to know but he could not give them real answers. He did not know. I had started being very snappy, pleasant one minute, horrible the next. He did not know if he was coming home to me still in my nightclothes, not washed, crying or smiling when he came in. Alternatively he might come in to find me wearing make-up, dressed, a meal on the table, with me brightly asking if he had had a good day. Poor Nick just never knew from one night to the next what it was going to be like and neither did I. My absence was also causing problems because the supply teachers were proving to be unsuitable. Hence the other staff in our senior department were complaining and asking when would I be back. Surely she was better now? What was she playing at? If she was fit to be shopping at Marks and Spencer then why was she not at work? Was she just 'playing the system'?

I asked to see the health visitor at the clinic and told her that we were both still struggling. She suggested that she would put us down for the 'sleep clinic', an intensive few sessions with another trained health visitor to identify and solve the problems. This sounded ideal and I asked her to proceed with it. Dominic also had to have a hearing test as a follow-up to the meningitis scare but there were no problems. Feeling more hopeful again, I carried on with a few more outings that week and we bought Dominic a second-hand baby walker. He liked to sit in it but did not move it initially.

My brother's wife Annie, baby Brendan and her daughters Indra and Kerita arrived at my parents for Christmas. Kevin could not get a ticket until a week or two later. My mother was worried how she could entertain them whilst she was at work and so I offered to take them to the various church groups I went to. Annie was a strong churchgoer in Zimbabwe and I thought she would like to be involved here. However, their arrival worried me as I irrationally felt 'Mum and Dad aren't going to help me now; that's it, they've gone. Dominic can't go there if they've got all these people. I've got to do it all myself now.' My parents had been helping out an awful lot, as much as they could. Yet we found that even if they had Dominic for a night, not only did they suffer from the resulting tiredness but also it would take us three nights to settle him back here. If he woke three times a night it was good going.

I began to really panic about silly things like what to have for our evening meal and worry all day about it. I started not wanting to answer the phone, which for me was unheard of. Whenever Dominic did sleep in the day, I then would be running round like a scalded cat, straightening the cushions and fanatically tidying up. I had to keep up appearances to prove I was coping. Meanwhile I felt the constant pressure as each sick note expired that I would have to go back to work soon. This terrified me but I began to chant to myself 'You've got to go back to work, you've got to go back to work' as I manically did needless chores.

The head teacher kept coming out to see me and because I could present a faked, confident exterior she probably felt justified in asking me when I intended returning. I would chatter on again about how I wanted to go back but inside I was absolutely crumbling and just thinking 'What's happened to my world? It's falling apart around me.' After she left I would rock myself, crying and yelling about school, 'I can't cope with it. I just don't want to know, I just can't handle this. I can't cope with me, how can I cope with teaching as well? It's not because I'm useless, it's not because I can't cope.' I did not know what it was.

As the end of term was approaching and she was getting hassled by the problems my absence was creating, she phoned me one day and said, 'You've been off a long time now and maybe it is time to take the first steps to returning to work. I would rather you came back and tried than not at all.'

Calmly I said I would maybe try it, even though my GP was still saying I was not ready. I then flung myself into complete panic, with her words ringing in my head all the time. I misinterpreted them as meaning 'I've got to go back, I've got to go back, and I've got to go back. I'll fail, I'll fail, but I've got to go back.' This sent me further round in circles and suddenly I turned it the other way, 'Right, I can cope. I'll do it, I'll do it.' What little energy I had left went into overdrive with an unnatural determination to succeed. With a stubborn self-defence I actually destroyed what was left of my sanity.

Instead of accepting that it did not matter if the house was a mess or if I did not get dressed, I went into overdrive trying to do it all. 'Right, if I've got to go back, I can do everything, but I'll have to stay up all night!' was my new motto. So I developed my night-time habits further. Dominic was now back sleeping in his nursery and I was in the small bedroom with the rest of the house at my disposal. I was dusting at half past two. I was in our study at three in the morning doing Christmas cards. I was ironing at four in the morning. I might have had two or three hours' sleep but lied to Nick that I had slept for much longer. Why sleep, as when I did Dominic would just wake me up? An irrational urgency built up in me to do the daily and seasonal chores – get the tree up and do this and do that. I covered my tracks by saying I had done the tasks during the day. All the time the threat 'you've got to go back, got to go back' ran around my head and I got more and more bitter about it.

I had continued with the postnatal depression support group but each week I just seemed to sink lower and lower. Others in the group felt it was good for them, but I just sat there like a reluctant teenager in a chemistry class. Bit by bit I felt myself sliding and falling, but talking was not saving me. I felt that it was something inside me which no amount of analysing, thinking, rationalising and trying to be logical could sort. To me, everything had taken an illogical turn. Normally in life I find if I have a problem I do something about it if I can. With this, no matter what I tried to do, I was getting blank walls. Earlier in the course I had been appalled when they appeared to let a fellow suffer leave after saying she felt suicidal, and I felt they let me down too at the last session. I was in tears and told them, 'I know the whys, the wherefores, possible reasons for this so-called illness, but I just can't seem to cope with *anything* now. I do not want to go out anymore. I'm not sleeping. I'm taking antidepressants, but I don't think they are helping. Everything seems to be falling apart and I've got to go back to work. I've got to go back, even if I fail, and I can't, but I've got to, I've got to, I've got to. Please help me.'

It was the end of our allotted time. End of session. Goodbye.

I felt all the pressures surrounding me, real or imaginary, were making me sink. Nobody would really say to me, 'Look, this will take time. You need help to relieve some of these pressures. Let's see what we can do.' I had the pressure from work, to go back to school. We needed my salary or we would lose the house we had worked so hard on. I had the pressure from my son, who demanded everything from me and did not sleep. I had the pressure from Nick, because obviously he was getting problems caused by me at work. He was trying so hard to make everything normal and wanted me to shake out of it and get on with our lives. I had the pressure from all my other friends who had got babies. A couple of those were also teachers and had successfully returned to work. I had the pressure still of finding suitable care for that baby whilst I went back to work. I had pressure from myself – why, why couldn't I do it all? I was angry with 'me' and at times wanted to hit myself. Everyone else copes with working and a baby. If I did go out now I would get the usual comment, 'Oh, I'm surprised you're not managing, it's not like you.' I had a total battering, felt from every direction.

The weekend after Dominic's christening he was very hot, miserable and sick again. By the Sunday afternoon we were all getting very worried about him and then debated long and hard if we should seek medical advice. Two days of paracetamol had not worked and I could not face another worrying night. A doctor did come to see him early evening, by which time he had brightened up considerably and smiled and gurgled without a care in the world. I was furious with this dreadful baby – how dare he make me look like an idiot? He too was obviously plotting against me. He had done since he was born. For the first time I felt I physically wanted to hit him.

Nick did not go to work again for a few days. He was ashen but seemed more concerned about me. He insisted on accompanying me as I went for a few Christmas presents. 'Huh, I cannot even do that now,' I thought. As it was the final Alpha class we both went – both skivers, obviously. The last few sessions of this had been wasted on me as just being with a group of six people now scared me. All I did was watch the clock and count the minutes until I could escape from all these people who knew I was a failure. God? What is he? Who is he? No matter who he was, he too would not want me. I was useless, but I had to go back to work. Go back and fail or not at all. Go back, go back.

Dominic began to master his baby walker and managed his first 'come to Mummy' by pushing his feet and reaching out to me across the kitchen floor in it. He was being cruel again, I thought, charming now but he would be awful in a few hours again. And I've got to go back to work. I did take Annie and Brendan to Mums and Tots but I hated being there. Too many people. Too high ceilings. Too noisy. People wanting to talk to me. Go away, go away. Cathy holding that baby who lived in our house. Oh, just keep him, keep him.

Back to sanity again, I demanded that Nick take some photographs of Dominic wearing his Christmas suit to send as festive cards. He obliged to try to please me, but Dominic refused to co-operate. Luckily Nick came up with the good idea to try him in his baby walker – it worked a treat and we had a roll of appropriate smiling pictures. We went to bed feeling much better but then struggled from 2.50 a.m. to 4.30 a.m. with a baby who refused to settle in any way and just cried and cried. Me too.

Luckily the next morning the 'sleep clinic' health visitor arrived. She suggested that we keep a sleep diary for the next week from which she could then help us to recognise any patterns or possible reasons. Her sympathetic manner and suggestions were appreciated and motivated us both that it would improve. Nick put up our Christmas lights above the garage and I collected the photographs of Dominic and put them into the cardholders for our family and closest friends. Sunday was better too. I went to church successfully with Dominic; we visited Granny H and he had his first white chocolate finger. He even 'danced' to a theme tune on the television and showed off his new trick of making 'clicks' with his tongue, giggling when we copied him. Even in the bath he laughed and kicked his legs excitedly. Meanwhile we wrote down every nap he had.

Nick felt and looked better so returned to school for the Christmas festivities. I coped with taking Dominic to our church coffee morning and took Annie and Brendan. Later he stayed with my mother whilst I saw my GP. On the previous visit she had asked me to write down for this appointment how I was and if I had any queries. I made this actual list:

1 Breast-feeding? Should I stop it? Will this finally break him away from me? I am reluctant to give Dominic a bottle – he is not keen either, therefore it restricts us both.
2 The pill? Could the mini-pill I am taking (needlessly, as passion does not exist in our house now) be affecting my moods?
3 Negative feelings about most things.
4 Mood swings with no logic.
5 Coping in general some days, but not many.
6 Fears and panics in crowds/people, especially theatre, at Mum's if there are lots of people there. Panic attacks – feels like I am late for something yet I may be just watching television or talking to someone.
7 Work: I have visited but felt scared. Feel pressure to return. I have read that many professional women who have suffered from PND do eventually go back to work, so why can't I?
8 Feelings that I want to harm Dominic and myself have begun to emerge.
9 More counselling? Will this help?
10 Exhausted: disturbed nights. Unable to sleep when Dominic does, day and night.
11 Relax: cannot.
12 I make arrangements to keep busy/cheer myself up then worry about silly details.
13 Headaches: above and behind eyes, varied frequency and intensity.
14 Anxiety: always seem to be thinking/worrying about things. I relive the birth/hospital, etc. I worry about silly household chores, e.g. what is for lunch.
15 Tearful: least thing or even nothing sets me off.
16 Relationships: Dominic – fine and I don't feel he is suffering. If I begin to want to harm him and/or myself, I'll ask for help and relief.
17 Nick: being supportive but I worry about tiredness – problems due to the meningitis drug and the pill.
18 Close relatives: want and need their help but on a very short fuse with them.
19 Friends: hurt if they don't enquire but then very touchy if they do!'

I also told her that I felt my biggest concern was pressure of time – fighting all the time to 'be normal' and panic that I had only got one or two weeks to get Dominic sleeping better and on the bottle. Then the thought of work terrified me as I could not cope with daily life yet, and I feel very guilty about it. My GP read the list and commented on aspects she could. We decided that with the sleep clinic help, it might lead to more sleep which would be a great asset. She increased my medication level and suggested that she should sign me off for at least six more weeks. This would give them a chance at school to plan a little more and hopefully give me the time to recover. I came away with mixed feelings, but decided to try to enjoy Christmas which was rapidly approaching.

All the mother and baby groups were having their parties that week so I took Dominic along with his auntie and cousin Brendan. I found it all very hard work but persevered. Dominic could at least sample bits of real food now and quite enjoyed munching on pieces of bread and fruit. My brother Kevin had now arrived back in England and my parents' house was very full. Brendan was a good baby who slept well and they could not understand why we were struggling so much. Currently Dominic had started another cold but in general that week his sleep pattern was a bit better. Our sleep clinic lady was pleased and felt we had all made progress that week. Why did I not feel it then?

We saw more friends that week too, such as Jeannie and Oliver. She looked great and had no problems with her handsome little baby. Dominic did actually sit up by himself that week for a few seconds. I could not understand why everyone seemed so pleased about it. We put up the Christmas tree, a task that normally delights me as I drink a glass of sherry and play Christmas music. Not this year. I only did it because it was expected of us. Dominic was sleeping more but I was hardly sleeping at all. I simply could not stop my mind from whirling between sensible thoughts about Christmas presents to the chant again of 'got to go back, got to go back. I'm a failure, useless failure'.

Another Monday dawned and with it Nick phoned in sick again. We must have been getting a terrible reputation by now. In the past Nick hardly ever had time off, often having 100% attendance, but not this year. I was too tired to go to our local Christmas coffee morning and also gave our apologies to my antenatal group as they too were meeting today. I began to rant about having no food in the house so we left Dominic with Kevin and his family whilst I insisted we shopped. So what if people saw us. Everyone knew by now that we were both just skiving. I did not care anymore. All the Christmas goods which normally delighted me just annoyed me this season. Bah humbug to it all.

For years I had kept a Christmas card given to me by my parents when I was about ten. The picture was a delicately painted version of baby Jesus lying in a manger. So often I had looked at this card over the years that followed, dreaming of a time when I too would have a beautiful baby. A child's first Christmas was something I had always anticipated for years. Last December, as a pregnant woman, I had fantasised about being able to buy a pink or blue 'baby's first Christmas' bauble for our tree. Those dreams were now tarnished and tattered, smashed on the floor like a broken bauble. Why had it all gone wrong? Why had I lost that loving feeling for my baby, my husband, my family, my friends, for myself? Festive spirit? You must be joking, now I knew why so many people hated Christmas.

After another very disturbed night, Dominic was very hot, miserable and clingy again. Nick too was getting very fed up of these spells and said that he would come to the surgery with me to see if we could get any answers. No luck. Yet again later on he was sick and I was up most of the night with him. How I wanted him to be quiet but to no avail. Next morning Nick decided he had better go to school. Staffing my class was a problem and if he was not in either, it created more problems. When he left I remember thinking that I felt in a good mood. I could tell the minute I woke up if it was a reasonable day or just a 'can I go back and just forget this day' sort of feeling. I was fine. I pottered around for a while. Eventually I took Dominic upstairs and decided to get us both dressed. As I walked upstairs I felt like a tidal wave was crashing down on us as this utter wave of exhaustion came over me. I panicked and I thought, 'I need to sleep, and I need to sleep now.' I put Dominic in his cot and pleaded with him, 'Please go to sleep Dominic.' But he had only recently woken up. I sobbed, 'I've got to sleep, I've got to sleep.'

Of course Dominic did not sleep and he started crying and crying and crying and crying. I just lay on the landing, at the top of the stairs, looking at the ceiling thinking, 'I can't go in to him, I'll hurt him if I go in there.' Suddenly I remembered one of the things that my first husband used to say to me, 'Children ruin your life.' That thought came and hit me smack in the face. He was right, and it was my fault for having him and I had brought this on myself.

Meanwhile Dominic was screaming and screaming. At that point I really knew I would seriously hurt him if I went in. I needed help and I needed it now. So I phoned Nick at school only to hear his recorded voice on the answer phone. It was the school Christmas lunch and everyone was in the dining room. I pressed redial for an hour, rocking myself, tears flowing and still hearing Dominic hysterical in his cot. All I wanted was my Nick. No one else would do. Redial. Rock. Redial. Rock. Redial. Rock. It went on and on. Eventually our school secretary brightly answered the phone. I sobbed I needed Nick. When he came on the line I simply said, 'Get home now.'

By the time he came home I just screamed at him 'Get that thing out of our house!', meaning Dominic. He grabbed his son and a bag of his kit and took him to my parents.

When Nick came back I was still sitting rocking at the top of the stairs. I had not moved for three hours and just said, 'I want to sleep.' He virtually carried me into the small bedroom and covered me up. All afternoon I kept trying and trying and trying to sleep, but I just could not. I was rocking and rocking and rocking to soothe myself. Eventually, because I could not sleep I started knocking my head against the wall just to go to sleep.

'Someone take my brain out, someone take my brain away from me,' I screeched. I started thinking this is what the children do at school, rocking and banging their heads, and I thought 'I'm doing it now', but I just couldn't stop. Once I had got into that rhythm of smacking myself I found that by giving myself a pain of some kind, it eased my mind somehow. It gave me something to focus on so I hit it harder. Will it hurt more next time – whack! Nick came up as he heard the noise getting louder and was horrified to see me throwing my head at the wall.

'What on earth are you doing?' he cried.

'Nothing, can't sleep, I've got to go back to school. I've got to go back or else I'll fail.'

Then I started rambling and rambling. 'What's for tea? What's for tea? What's for tea? Ironing needs doing. Should I put the washing on? What shall I do?' I had totally flipped.

Nick got the doctor out to me. I was a ranting lunatic but as soon as the doctor arrived I thought, 'Help! Someone's here to help me. They'll put me to sleep' and I sat up. I was perfectly sensible and coherent within a split second. I said, 'Just give me an injection and put me to sleep please. I don't want to die, just turn my brain off for me please.'

'Well, I've no injections but I can leave you some sleeping pills,' he replied.

I had a couple of them and they just did not work. I did not go to sleep at all, and that made me even worse then because I thought, 'I can't get out of this trap.' My parents came. I could not bear them to touch me. My mother kept saying, 'Oh love, you just need a cuddle.'

'Don't touch me, get off me, get off me,' I yelled back.

My father kept trying different ways to shake me out of it and said, 'Oh come on now, you're being silly.' At that comment I whacked my head against the wall even harder and sunk my teeth into his hand. I was aware of all this but I just felt like I was watching it from the corner. This was not me, I do not know who it was. Again they got the doctor. He gave me some stronger sleeping pills to put me to sleep. These did work and as I felt myself float off it was pure heaven.

I remember I woke up at about midnight again, so they had only knocked me out for a matter of two or three hours. I was really annoyed as I felt he should have knocked me out for a day at least, but he did not. Nick was in bed asleep. Dominic was at my parents for the night. I went downstairs, made myself a milky drink and then sat in the chair in the nursery. It was dark and peaceful. Outside it was raining. Soft, gentle drops. I decided I wanted to go for a walk, as a walk in the rain could be soothing. I put my mug down and walked downstairs and out of the front door wearing just my nightdress. It was 19 December. I left the front door open and out I went. I just wandered all round the local streets and saw no one. I walked up to the church because I felt comfortable there and needed the peace that some of the parishioners held. I just sat in the doorway, crying and rocking, getting drenched. Then at one point I wondered if Nick had noticed I had gone, so went to look. You can see our house very clearly from the top of the hill. There was a police car outside, and I went to sit back down and thought 'Oh damn! Someone's coming for me.'

Eventually it was my brother and father who found me. When Nick had realised I was missing he had phoned the police and my parents who were all searching for me. My father had suspected for some reason that I might be at the church. I heard the car come up the drive and Kevin sprung out with obvious relief, declaring, 'There you are!'

He sat down beside me and put his arm around me without saying a word. When he did speak he just said how cold and wet I was and that we should go. I let him guide me into the back of our parents' car. My father was driving. They threw a blanket around me and I buried my head into Kevin's warm body and jumper. For some reason they did not bring me home to my Nick but back to my parents' house. I went more berserk because I knew I could not relax in there any more. My obsessive tidiness made me want to keep all my surroundings immaculate and at their house I felt that there was always something that needed doing. Nick and I are very tidy and with all the people staying at my parents', their house was the opposite. Tonight there was no way I would set foot in that house. I was yelling and screaming, 'Don't take me in that house, there's too much to do. There's too much to do and I can't do it all. There's too much, there's too much.'

As I was ranting and screaming two policemen appeared in the driveway holding batons just in case I became violent with them. I vaguely remember someone telling them that I would be fine and thanking them for their involvement. They left and I was brought back home. They gave me some more sleeping pills. A second police team came and again checked I was all right.

I had some more sleeping tablets. They put me back to bed with Nick upstairs. My father was in the front bedroom and my mother was in the other spare bedroom, as they thought we needed more help. Meanwhile poor Annie was struggling through the night with a very upset Dominic. I woke up at six o'clock, 'ping!', wide awake and I had this dreadful urge to hurt myself. I went downstairs, got the big block of knives off the side in the kitchen, and set to making patterns in my legs with all the knives. Nick came down to find me with blood running down my legs, stabbing at myself and muttering that these knives were blunt. My parents appeared too and all three were guilt ridden that they had not heard me. They put me back upstairs to bed and I assured them I would be fine. As soon as I was left alone this yearning for self-harm emerged and I spent the next few hours attacking myself with anything appropriate in the room. I took a photograph frame apart and cut my face with it. I put my hand round the light bulbs and burnt it. I stabbed my entire arm with scissors.

Every time Nick took something away from me he would stay with me until I was asleep again. I pretended to be asleep though, like a child, and then found something else to abuse myself with. By hurting myself I somehow found something else to focus on. That is all I could put it down to. As my mind was just in such a mush I could not logically think about anything. Eventually the psychiatrist came over from the local hospital. I talked to him but wanted to laugh because he was wearing open sandals in December. 'What a stupid man,' I thought. He called Nick into the room and said that in his opinion I did need a hospital stay until I was more stable. He explained that there was a mother and baby unit that I could go to for a couple of days, where Dominic could go with me and they could assess how I was really coping. I agreed to go. He phoned to check with the hospital and they said that they did not have the staff in for the mother and baby unit that day. The doctor decided that I did need admitting urgently so I would have to go for the first night on the ordinary ward and Dominic could join me the following day.

With this news I bounced out of bed, got myself washed and dressed. I excitedly packed my bags as though I were going on holiday. It was a week before Christmas and I was delighted to be 'checking in' at the area's renowned psychiatric hospital. I was going to the local Victorian asylum where everyone in the community joked about being sent. Now, should I pack my Swiss Army knife this time?

CHAPTER 14

A refuge

On the 25-minute journey to the psychiatric hospital, I actually felt excited! I doubt if this was how Nick was feeling. I chatted incessantly about how I would be fine after a couple of days and that by Christmas, which was only six days away, all would be well. The hospital was a huge old Victorian asylum which had been used as a war hospital and subsequently as a psychiatric hospital for the area. It could be seen for miles due to its distinctive tower in the centre and had many two- and three-storey wings for wards. At its prime it was a huge community and had its own chapel, gardens and many outbuildings and facilities. In recent years, with the introduction of care in the community, its wards were now mainly empty and in disrepair as its total closure and demolition were imminent during the next few months. Now the site is an executive home residential area. It was in the same village where Nick had grown up and where his family still lived. As a child he had regularly played in the grounds and even cycled around the vast corridors on his bicycle! Now he was bringing his wife to be admitted.

We parked at the main entrance. Nick grasped my hand and carried my bag in the other and we walked up the steps of the main entrance. A security guard nodded at us and asked if he could help. Nick mentioned the ward number and duly was given directions. The corridor of the main entrance was bright and carpeted, with plenty of notice boards and a few displays of the newer, smaller hospitals that would replace it. A few office staff carried out their business. It was initially welcoming. As we turned into the main corridors the change was dramatic. They were deserted. They seemed cold with the classic white and green tiled walls. The sound of our footsteps echoed as we searched for the appropriate sign. In the distance a door banged shut. For a moment all the horrific scenarios of asylums flooded my mind and I felt I was walking amongst the ghosts of shrieking, tormented souls running down those corridors in voluminous, filthy white gowns. It reminded me also of a favourite poem of mine about silence that suggests that the totally silent places are those 'where man hath been' in the past. My heart was pounding and my grasp on Nick's hand tightened as I suddenly felt worried. At that point we found the correct ward, one of the few still operating, and climbed the stairs to it.

Apparently the ward for our particular locality was full that evening so I was to be initially admitted for one night to an alternative ward upstairs, intended for patients from a different town than ours. I cannot remember the next few hours except for hearing a group of visiting carol singers in the ward, whilst we waited in a small side room. By early evening and after Nick had gone, I went to my bed. The lighting and décor of the ward made a warm, orange glow that seemed to soothe me. When a member of staff came to chat to me, I logically talked to her about the events leading up to my admittance. She listened and patted me on the leg and said that I had obviously been through a terrible time but they were there to help and they would make every attempt to do so. I wanted to hug her. Tactfully she asked if she could just have a little look in my bag for any sharp items and explained it was ward policy. She took a couple of things with her and left me to unpack my bag properly and settle in. I watched her walk out of the room and turned to my bag again. I stroked a small, white teddy bear of Dominic's that Nick had suggested I brought and buried my face in it for any sign of his aroma (just a little), and I briefly thought of his smiling face. I took out my nightdress and dressing gown and laid them on the bed. I then came to my toilet bag and, for some unknown reason, an overwhelming urge to hurt myself erupted from nowhere. It was like a huge surge of hunger that had to be sated. In a wild flurry I searched in vain for anything I could stab myself with. Toothbrush – no. Shampoo – no. Hairbrush – mm, made a dint but no good. Cleanser – rubbish. Emery board – ah, not bad but not good enough. In frustration I used my nails instead and a few minutes later the lovely nurse came back to find me sobbing hysterically and gouging my arms with my own fingernails.

She shouted for more help and immediately grabbed my wrists and sat with me, gently rocking and calming me. As silent tears rolled down my cheeks and I began to relax into the rhythm she had set, I did feel better and the crisis point had passed again. I apologised but she said there was no need and again reminded me that I was there to get better, but that they understood it would take time. She and another nurse then suggested I tried to sleep and helped me into my nightclothes and bed. Little by little other patients seemed to quietly appear and go to bed. I just kept my head down. I did not want to speak to anyone. I tried and tried again to sleep. Time passed by and the ward became darker and quiet. Still I could not sleep. I tried to rock myself back and forth to try to relax and to sleep, but it did not work. Gradually I began to get annoyed so kicked one of my shins with my other heel. Stupid body. If it would not relax, what else could I do with it? Kick, kick, rock. Still no sleep. Who cares? I don't. Kick, kick, bite. I sank my teeth into my forearm too. Eventually I was kicking, scratching, biting and throwing my head against the bedside table in a frenzied, self-abusing attack. Staff came running and I attacked them in my wild, distraught state. I tried to hit and bite them but it was just me I wanted to hurt. They were just in the way. I think there were about four or five people finally trying to hold me down safely. In the end I dissolved into tears and flopped. They gradually released their holds but I began again to strike out. At last the wave of violence did pass and I sank exhaustedly into a numb, shocked state, mumbling again that I did not want to die, I just wanted my brain switched off for a while. I wanted so much to sleep but I could not do so.

As staff retreated, the same good nurse gently took me by the hand and told me to go with her. Meanwhile her colleague took some blankets from my bed. They led me to the lounge area of the ward where they were based during night duty and settled me into a large, comfortable chair, swathed in blankets. Someone brought me a warm, milky drink and I cradled it in both hands. Little by little I sipped it until it was empty. The cup was taken from me and I was told I could stay as long as I wanted. For a few hours I sat with the staff as they knitted, chatted, embroidered and gossiped away on night duty. Occasionally someone would give me a smile and ask 'Okay?' I would nod and just relax again. I felt so humble and grateful to these people. Earlier I had been trying to head-butt them and now here I was listening to what Christmas presents they had bought for their auntie! Yet in those small hours of that December morning I felt some true calm and relaxation that I had not felt for months. It was the first glimmer of hope for recovery and just being allowed to sit, with no pressure in any way, was a terrific healing mechanism. Just as some of the night staff had let me sit with them in the maternity ward back in April, this approach was just what I needed at this stage too.

At last I said I thought I might be able to sleep so I was taken back to my bed. It had been remade in my absence and looked inviting – a small touch but important. The nurse took the blankets from my shoulders and tucked me up, stroking my forehead as she wished me sweet dreams. I slept until it was daylight and realised everyone else had been up for ages. I presume there had been instructions not to disturb me. The nurse who had been with me all along brought me a drink and some toast and said she was going off duty. She explained that I would be moving up to the correct ward later on and that she wished me well. One sense of disappointment I have still today is that I cannot even remember what this lady looked like, her name or anything other than the kindness she showed me. She and her colleagues were excellent in that ward and their patients were honoured to have them.

I dressed, which was expected during the day at this hospital, and packed my bag again. One of the new staff came into the ward and said she would take me down to where I was supposed to be, as there was now a bed available. I had to have two nurses to escort me down, presumably in case I struck out again. The first ward had been decorated in warm colours. Downstairs the first thing that occurred to me was how cold it appeared, everywhere painted with pale blue. I was told to sit at one of the tables in what appeared to be a dining area. One of the nurses who had brought me down attracted the attention of a member of staff on this ward, passed her a brown file, nodded in my direction, waved and left. The lady she had given the file to glanced at me and disappeared into a small room. I was left with my bags, sitting at a table. I was aware of other people sitting at other tables. I did not know who were the staff, patients or visitors. The absence of uniforms makes such places very confusing. Every now and then someone would appear from the small room but head off in every direction but mine. Amid the bustle of people, hum of conversations and a cleaner doing her job, I began to feel isolated and frightened. I wanted to rock myself but just stared at the table instead. The sounds around me seemed to get louder and louder and, as my fears grew, I felt I was falling into a huge hole. To 'save' myself I felt the urge to hurt myself rise again. Little by little, I began to dig my nails into the back of my hands. Where was someone? What were they doing leaving me here 'alone in a room full of strangers'. I smiled as I realised that was a cue for a song but immediately panicked and scratched more deeply. By the time someone did come to me my hands were bleeding.

The person noticed my hands, looked at them, tutted and told me it was a stupid thing to do. I was shown into a tiny room with three high-backed chairs and a table in it and told that someone would see me soon. I was left alone again. Eventually another lady came in and said that because I had done all this damage to myself and towards the staff, then consequently there was no way they could let the baby anywhere near me at the moment. She said that even if they did have the staff to cover the Mother and Baby unit they could not let me use it as it would not be safe for everyone concerned. In my current state of mind I did not care. I did not want to see Dominic. I did not want to see anybody. Once again I was left alone. I could hear some Christmas music playing somewhere. I hated it. I hated everything, especially me. In this bare room the only decoration was a small, plastic holly ornament on a solitary nail in the middle of a vast, pale blue wall. The door was slightly ajar. I snatched the holly off the wall, flung it out of the room and smacked my head against the naked wall. I pushed a chair out of the corner and crouched in the space it had been, rocking and sobbing.

At last I was aware someone was in the room. A brief glance up and I saw a young, smartly dressed man watching me. He asked me a few questions and I ignored him. In my head I was using swear words I hardly knew, let alone use. In the end I did swear at him to mind his own business. I do not swear normally. Once, as a teenager, I did use the 'f' word for effect with some of the 'in' girls in my class. They were amazed but laughed at me because they said it did not suit me. I felt so uncomfortable and embarrassed that I rarely did it again! Yet here I was swearing at a doctor. Meanwhile he read through my notes and eventually sighed.

'Well,' he said. 'You've proved your point, you're not well. Now you can either sit and talk to me properly, or not. What's it going to be? We know you need help. We're here to help, but we can't help you with all this going on. I know you are not stupid. You are an intelligent woman. I want to talk and listen to you, but I would much rather you sat in one of these empty chairs and looked at me.'

This approach did work and slowly I moved and curled up in this big, uncomfortable chair. Maybe, had there been an inviting sofa and cushions there in the first place, I would have used them. Big chairs meant for the elderly were not ideal in such a room.

At last I did begin to talk to him about all the build-up to my admittance and my desperate need for sleep. He agreed and said he would write me up a prescription for some sleeping pills and stronger antidepressants. He said that they would not work immediately but we would have to see how I went on. I would be allowed home a little if I wanted to go but he suggested that I did need some time with them in hospital. By the end of the session I felt much better and he called in a lady who was to be my named nurse and we all confirmed the decisions that had been made. From there she took me to my bed, the first one in the ward, and once again I unpacked, in time for a look around before lunch.

The ward appeared to be like a small 'h' shape. The entrance to it at the top led down a corridor, with small rooms off it. This led onto the main hub of the ward behind a huge white door which was usually locked. This opened into the dining room with the kitchen, nurse's office and a small consultation room leading off it. It was all decorated for Christmas with a tree, lights and decorations. The dining area had about five round tables with chairs and also served as the visiting area. It always smelled of stale food. Just along from here was the lounge which looked like a nursing home with big, straight-backed chairs, a television and a couple of tables. On a couple of shelves were some jigsaw puzzles and battered games. There was a separate room between the main day areas for smokers. It was like a waiting room at a station – bare, yellow and smelly with a few old and tatty magazines strewn around. At either end of the main areas were the two bedrooms and bathrooms. Each patient had their own bed, wardrobe and bedside cabinet. There were no curtains dividing the beds. The furniture was used for privacy. I estimate each room had about ten beds in it. There was only one single bedroom.

I was aware that it was lunchtime by other patients making their way into the dining room and all other areas immediately becoming quiet. The food was served from a hatch into the kitchen, but initially a trolley was brought into the dining area with six big metal teapots and some bread and butter for each table. As I learnt later, some patients had laid the tables earlier and appeared to have their own places. I did not know where to sit so queued for my food, picked up a knife and fork and sat at a table on my own. There seemed to be no staff around other than one who was assisting an elderly lady with her meal. I felt shy and scared. The food felt like lumps in my dry mouth. Luckily, from one table a friendly voice informed me that there was room on their table. I joined four other ladies who were to become my meal 'friends' for several weeks to come. Hardly anyone spoke other than to ask how much sugar to put in their tea. Three of my fellow diners were elderly and other than appearing to be a bit confused and slow, seemed fine to me (yet I probably did to them). The other lady was middle-aged, very gentle and quiet with piercing eyes, as if she were trying to tell you something that you could not understand.

Usually in hospital your relationship with other patients develops very quickly as you chat about your respective reasons for being there and discuss your family, job and life in general. In the early days in the ward, none of these topics seemed to arise. Conversation was based around meal-times and the strength of the tea. I did not want to communicate and neither did anyone else it seemed. None of the staff seemed to want to chat either. I wanted to talk at times but no one was around to listen.

Nick arrived at some stage and told me about what had happened at home. He had not gone back into school due to my situation and with it being the last few days before Christmas his assistants would be managing the festivities for his class as necessary. Dominic had spent most of the time at my parents since I had become so ill. Claire had now joined the swelling numbers there and he was amused and cared for by a team of relative strangers other than my parents. Nick would collect him in between visits to me and take him home for a while.

During my first afternoon on the correct ward Nick also spoke to staff and everyone agreed that the initial suggestion of both Dominic and I being admitted to the Mother and Baby ward was not viable. I also started on my first tablets of the new medication. By teatime I felt a little happier as at least I knew where to sit and actually enjoyed my meal and cup of tea. At each mealtime a nurse would bring in the medication trolley and we would wait to be called up for our own. I felt myself getting excited at the prospect of walking up for mine but at the same time almost scared of others watching me. So few of us had eye contact with anyone on the way back to our place. It was amazing how quickly I felt swallowed into institu-tionalisation. By early evening visitors left and most people went through to the lounge area or smoking room. There was another drinks trolley at nine o'clock for patients. Visitors had to use a vending machine. The live-liest area did seem to be the smokers' room for both staff and patients. I almost felt I wanted to smoke to be part of it. Instead I sat with some of the elderly ladies in the big chairs watching television. I began to feel very restless and if I tried to relax my legs would jerk. One elderly lady caused the staff a great deal of work as she constantly shouted out, would complain loudly about everything and generally took up more attention than the rest of us put together. She was put in the only single room quite early on for the night, but she still shouted spasmodically. I realised that it was getting to be bedtime for us all as the patients suddenly seemed to put on their nightclothes and assemble in the dining area again. Not wishing to be left out I did the same. The ritual was a bedtime drink and medication. As I held my cup my arm twitched and I spilt some – odd, I thought. Shortly we all wandered off to our respective beds but I felt far from sleepy.

Once again I found myself in a darkened room but could not settle at all. Also, I was beginning to feel very full and uncomfortable with my milk-laden breasts and no baby to release the pressure. I like to sleep on my front but with these hard 'footballs' it was impossible. Gradually the sound of snores, fidgeting and other bodily noises filtered through the darkness. I felt the start of a self-mutilation urge, so got up to find a member of staff. Maybe if I had another drink it would help. I wandered back towards the dining area but could find no one. Eventually one of the staff appeared. She was a large woman with short hair and masculine features. She was abrupt with me and sharply asked what was I doing out of bed. I explained that I could not settle and wondered if I could talk to someone and have a milky drink. In a nasty tone of voice she told me that there were no drinks available at this time of night and that the main kitchen only sent them a certain amount each evening and there was none left. She suggested I went back to bed again. Like a scared child I ran back to my bed and resisted the urge to hurt myself again but lay there twitching uncontrollably. Now what was wrong with me? I kept trying to imagine the previous night and how calm I had felt wrapped in a blanket. I had suffered at night for months and being confined to bed was torture. The night passed by bearably for me due to the commotion, several hours later, of the admission of an alcoholic whose children had found her passed out on the kitchen floor. Various staff and her family members seemed to spend ages talking in angry voices to her, saying they were fed up with the number of times 'she had been in this place' and that this time should be the last. It was sad that someone else's illness helped me through a bad night.

I think I did manage a couple of hours' sleep. After breakfast I had a pleasant surprise with a visit from our vicar. I was genuinely glad to see him and due to his position he was allowed into the lounge area. We sat and held hands as we talked and I found him a great comfort. It was to be the first of many visits to me and I appreciated his compassion and friendship at such a difficult time. Although I cannot remember specifically what we talked about, I know his very presence did calm me and gave me hope that one day I would be well again. That morning I also received a beautiful bouquet from the school staff. I remember feeling at bit upset when I asked a nurse for a vase. I arranged them but was stopped from putting them at my bedside. I was told that flowers stayed in the lounge for everyone to enjoy. Yet they were for me and I felt entitled to be selfish.

Later on I was upset with my sore, heavy breasts and asked a couple of staff for advice. All one heavily-busted woman commented was that I should be grateful that it would be short-lived as she was saddled with a big pair all the time! Luckily another lady was more sympathetic and managed to get me some painkillers which helped a little. Gradually the pressure did ease over the next week or so.

Nick visited in the afternoon and I gave him washing for home. We began 'Hanzak lists' for items between hospital and home and such aspects of domesticity formed part of the visiting routine. I told him about my limbs twitching and sore breasts but also that I did feel a bit better. That evening he brought my mother and Dominic briefly to see me. I really did not want to see them for some unknown reason and a few minutes was enough. Nick wrote in Dominic's diary that he was pleased to see me though. Months later I was pleased to see how Nick had continued the diary in my absence, noting at this point that Dom, as we now called him sometimes, had developed a funny laugh, especially at night. He also sucked his gums, made strange faces and was getting better at trying to sit up.

My second night on this ward was awful. Once again we were sent to bed and an eerie stillness grew around the ward. Where did the staff go at night? The twitching grew worse and worse. I did feel like I could sleep that night, but physically when I did relax my limbs would jerk violently. I became more and more distressed and no one seemed to visit the ward. I got up and wandered around the lounge area, trying to see if I could settle better after that. The same night nurse was on duty again and sent me back to bed. I told her the problem but she said to try to forget about it. I tried and tried to relax but presumably as the sleeping tablet took a little effect I was semi-sedated and got out of bed again, wandering with my twitching limbs. I was confused, dazed and very, very scared. I wandered like a drunk around the deserted rooms and eventually collided with a tall bookcase. I split my lip and banged the side of my face. I was aware of a crash and then a bright light going on. It was that same abrupt nurse again! I had knocked a potted plant off the bookcase and it was lying smashed and shattered all over the floor. The nurse angrily shouted at me, called me a troublemaker and said she had predicted that I would be a problem. The rest of the night I cowered under my covers like a naughty child, too terrified to move, apart from the spasmodic jerks. At the time I did not consider what effect her attitude had upon me, but with hindsight it was very damaging.

I was so relieved to see the day staff and hoped that the next night would be better. I told Nick about my terrible night when he came the next day. I saw him tell my 'named nurse' who apparently checked the notes and no mention had been made of it. I felt they both thought I was lying and yet I knew I was right. Fine, if they do not believe me, I thought, then I will just have to carry on myself. If they think the medication should make me sleep then I must be failing again, so tonight I will make it work for sure.

I had a surprise visit from Nick's friends that day who were en route to see relatives in Liverpool. As it was not true visiting time, they let me see them in the small consultation room. I vaguely remember wittering about many things to them. The wife of the couple said something which I interpreted to imply that she could not understand what was wrong with me, as I now had everything I wanted. I freaked out and yelled at her. I climbed onto her husband's lap, asking him for a hug and generally behaved very strangely. I was not well enough to see them.

That night another nurse found me curled up in a dark corner of the ward, sobbing silently, rocking and digging holes out of my fingers with my thumbnails. Every now and then I would mumble 'Too scared ... I'm trouble ... too scared'. She asked what I was doing and when I explained about the unbearable twitching but I was frightened to ask for help, she did at least hug me, put me back into bed and reassured me that it must be the new medication which was not suiting me. Immediately I felt better knowing that there was a reason for it. I had begun to feel that I was doing it myself subconsciously. Maybe it was another part of my lunacy. To be believed, given an explanation and reassured was a great help and I was able to settle better. She even put some plasters on my bleeding fingers.

The following day was Christmas Eve and doctors were in short supply. By lunchtime I was very worried that my medication was not changed and it took Nick's demands before a locum doctor was asked to take action. Within hours the twitching had eased to a bearable level. The ward had become very quiet as all patients, where possible, had gone home for Christmas and staffing levels had been reduced. By Nick's second visit that day I was much better. He said he had left Dominic at his mother's and suggested, after a chat with the staff, that I should go out for a visit there for half an hour. Hesitantly I did so. I had only been in hospital a few days but already the 'outside world' seemed to be a huge challenge. I was able to slip into 'I'm fine' mode at my mother-in-law's, but after a drink wanted to go back to the ward. It felt surrealistic. I did not know who or what I was at this stage. I felt secure back on the ward and felt no emotion at seeing Dominic leave. I always felt sorry to see Nick go.

It was sad that on Dominic's first Christmas morning he was without his parents. Although his grandparents and relatives were doing well with him, physically he looked pathetic on Christmas Day photographs. His face had big red patches of eczema that had flared up and he looked quite lost and bewildered. Meanwhile I woke up on the ward with no excitement whatsoever. Normally I am still a big kid about everything associated with the season – not this year. However, Nick collected me and we went to his mother's for lunch. All the photographs of that visit mainly show Nick, Granny H and Dominic. I opted out and just took them. The most effective present was a singing and dancing pig which fascinated Dominic, until it made him cry! He received many presents from the family and our friends. All I had got for him was a cassette player we had bought at Rutland Water, in the summer. Lunch passed off well and we decided to call at our house prior to going to my parents'. It was my first visit home. As Dominic needed changing, I offered to do it and took him up to his room. He began to cry. I took his nappy off. He cried. I wiped him. He cried. I put a clean nappy on. He cried. I put on his trousers. He cried. I picked him up. He cried. I shook him. He cried. I shook and shook him. He cried. Luckily Nick came in and grabbed him from me, asking, 'What are you doing?'

Numbly, I replied I was shaking 'that noisy bag of bones to shut it up'. I felt nothing but the desire to stop that noise. That noise which had disturbed me for so long. That noise which had ruined me.

From there Nick debated if he should take me straight back to hospital. I said I would be fine if the noise did not start again. So we had a buffet meal at my parents' house with my side of the family. I felt like a stranger, as if I were not there. I was just watching a film, detached and cold. I smiled for photographs and opened presents. Physically I was there but mentally I was nowhere, just a shadow of my former self. Back at the hospital I wandered happily to my bed and Nick had to report on my behaviour during the day. The incident of me shaking Dominic led to him being placed on the 'at risk' register. Happy Christmas!

So by the end of Dominic's eighth month he had been christened, had his first Christmas, met Father Christmas for the first time and been placed on the 'at risk' register by social services! His typical day was spent with his African cousins, at Christmas parties and using his baby walker and bouncer. He weighed 20 lb 9 oz and was 72 cm long. His bedtime was varied; his sleep and daily pattern non-existent but he could sit up unaided. He had been having feeds from his mother three times a day but now was totally on formula milk with some solids, especially white chocolate fingers. He could make clicking noises with his tongue and liked playing with crinkly paper. Yet the biggest event was that he had been separated from his mother, now in a hospital for the mentally ill. What a month!

CHAPTER 15

Becoming institutionalised

A few days after Christmas I had sickness and diarrhoea, blamed on the next lot of medication! They then had to try another drug. I had begun to sleep a little better and had moved bed position in the ward. I now was down at the bottom next to a wall. I liked this space as I felt secure but not far from other people. The days began to merge and I drifted from one mealtime and drink to the next. I saw Nick daily but not much of Dominic. I still did not want to see most of my family in hospital, but asked for a few of my friends to pop in. I liked them coming and it gave Nick a break. Not long before Kevin and his family were due to fly back to Zimbabwe, I complained that he had not been to see me. Nick had to remind me that I had requested not to see any of them! People I normally loved and whose company I cherished, I somehow pushed away. Maybe it was the look of pain and worry in their eyes I could not handle. I did not want sympathy or love. I did not know what I wanted.

I had received letters in Christmas cards from some of my college friends, as usual. This year though I replied immediately to two of them who were now also mothers. I found it therapeutic to write about what had happened and wrote volumes to them about my thoughts and fears. They wrote back and for a few weeks played a strong role in my recovery. Sue has since reminded me that I also wrote a very long letter to her at this time, explaining what had happened to me over the previous weeks. I signed it 'from someone who used to be Elaine'.

Although the twitching had subsided and my stomach had settled, at times I still had the dreadful urge to harm myself. With time I was allowed more at my bedside and yet I still hurt myself. I used the cassette box from the tapes I had asked Nick to bring in for me. Staff had suggested I might relax listening to favourite music on a Walkman, usually Lionel Richie. When I did feel ready for a photograph of Dominic, a day or two later I took the frame apart and slashed at my arm with it. One day another patient showed me scars all over her body from self-abuse. I was actually sitting on the toilet at the time! The locks were non-existent, and she just pushed the door open and sat on the floor to tell me her history! It was not an environment in which to be prudish or vain. There were few mirrors on the ward because they had been smashed and used for abusive purposes. One night I overheard the repercussions of this patient's latest attack on herself as they waited for an ambulance for her. Staff chastised her for wasting everyone's time and said 'A and E' at the general hospital had better things to do than patch up people like her repeatedly. Once upon a time I might have agreed with them, but having experienced these urges you are powerless to stop yourself and obviously do need help, not criticism, to prevent it happening again.

My fear of the nurse who had scared me so much in my early nights never really left me. Maybe her manner during those nights was due to other problems she had, but nonetheless they were not good nursing qualities. I was very vulnerable and did not need shouting at. However, I did begin to feel more secure with myself on the ward and became more talkative. Staff often apologised about the lack of activities and said it was due to the Christmas season but also, due to their forthcoming closure, many services were being moved elsewhere. I spent New Year's Eve initially with a visit from my parents, then with my fellow elderly patients. We watched the film 'Shadowlands' until the usual medication and drink trolley time, then went off to bed. We were disturbed by the admission of another alcoholic at four o'clock. I was awake then for four hours and had just drifted off when I was sharply told by a nurse that I must get up. 'What for?', I wondered. The only purpose I could see was that I should phone Nick and ask him to come and rescue me! He did so later on and I came home for a cuddly, relaxed afternoon with him.

During this period Nick found me very difficult to talk to because of my enormous mood and personality swings. One moment I seemed to gain confidence and stability and the next I seemed illogical, confused and angry. I was confused about why I was in hospital yet at the same time knew I could not deal with life outside the institution. I was angry that my medication was always being changed and not seeming to have any settling effect. Other than the drugs, I felt I was not having any other treatment or counselling that I felt I needed. However, Nick pointed out that we had already had lengthy discussions with a psychiatrist and senior nursing staff as to the reasons why I was there and why I should stay for the time being. Some visits I was emotional and upset, questioning why this had happened to me. My initial experiences with some of the staff on this ward had made me wary, uncertain and hesitant as to how much trust I could put in them. Consequently I did not bond with them and it was up to Nick on his visits to relay any problems, concerns or worries I had. Yet on the rare occasions I had to chat to a nurse willing to listen to me, I would feel in a high and happy mood afterwards. Initially I was not interested in details of Dominic or my family but would only talk about the ward happenings and the other patients and staff. Gradually I was becoming further alienated from everything that had been normal for me. During one consultation with the main psychiatrist, Nick asked if they had decided what my actual condition was. He told us that it was likely to be the most severe form of postnatal depression – puerperal psychosis – which can affect about two in 1000 women after birth. They gave us leaflets to read about it but generally we had little information to help us.

From Boxing Day, Nick had kept Dominic at home every night for stability, and also as my parents' household was struggling enough with the rest of the family without a crying baby disturbing them all every night too. This put greater pressure on Nick as then he was having disturbed nights and stressful days both with his son and wife! He survived by facing each day at a time and concentrating on the practicalities of childcare and hospital visiting. He organised each day for Dominic between himself, the grandparents and Cathy, with only the occasional and short visit between mother and son. When he did come I apparently could not hold him due to the worries of me harming him and he would stay in his car seat. Equally I did not really want to fuss him and was very cold towards him. In his diary it is noticeable that when Dominic had seen me he was upset that night at home. Ironically the advice in his diary at this point is that the mother should make time for herself, but I do not think it meant this extreme. The poor little mite must have been very confused. He did please Nick by learning to sit up in the bath and splash even more. Occasionally Dominic would sleep through for his father, or only wake once, so he was settled to a certain extent.

At one stage we were shown around the Mother and Baby unit. It was accessed by a staircase just outside my ward. It had a couple of bedrooms, kitchen, bathroom and lounge areas, all equipped with a range of baby toys and equipment. We were told that when in use it was staffed by two nurses, 24 hours a day, who served to monitor the mother with her child and assist where necessary. The aim was to help their bonding relationship and to teach the mother parenting skills and coping strategies. Currently the general decision regarding me using it was that I still needed to be helped to get better before I could even begin to build a relationship with my son. I was not functioning as an individual myself so I could go no further at this point.

On a relatively good day, Nick might suggest a trip out and sometimes I would agree. Consequently I decided to try a visit home the first Sunday of the new year. I noticed that Dominic had learnt to clap his hands but I was more interested in bits of post and choosing a few items to take back to hospital with me. I still felt cold towards him and hated any crying he made.

As the new year came and went the hospital did seem to be busier and I noticed some patients saw occupational and physiotherapists. Yet nothing much seemed to change for me. I had seen the same psychiatrist a few times and one morning Nick was asked to come in at a specific time for a chat with him. He arrived and I was told I had to see the doctor with him. Instead of going into the small consultation room as usual, we followed my named nurse down the corridor. She briefly said there were a few people to see us. The door opened and my psychiatrist invited us to sit down by the desk at which he was seated. My heart pounded though as there were about eight other people in there, all with files and papers on their laps, pens poised, staring at us. I was terrified. During the last weeks I had become more and more withdrawn from people and being faced by this sea of professionals absolutely horrified me. The doctor asked, 'Well, how are you?', but all I could think was, 'Who are all these people?' It would have been common decency to say who they were and why they should be involved with me. The only exception was one lady, a social worker who I had been at a case conference with for one of my pupils at school. But the rest? I presumed that they were students or whatever, but to me it was a very poor situation to be in. I could not concentrate on the questions being asked due to the panic that the presence of these other people was causing me.

The doctor proceeded to glance at his notes, ask me questions about how I had been feeling and make comments about my behaviour. At one point he said it was as if I had been copying pupils I had taught. He concluded that he and 'others' felt there was no more they could do for me and that he recommended I was discharged tomorrow. I could hardly believe my ears. Fighting back the tears, I said that I still had these terrible urges to hurt myself and I was worried what I might do to Dominic if I was allowed straight back home. He asked if I was threatening him. This made me feel worse and I mumbled that all I wanted was my life back. I had come here for help and if I could not get it, I really did not know what to do. I began to cry and mumbled, 'What? What? I can't go home.'

'I'm only following the recommendations of the previous doctor', he replied.

This other doctor had seen me once and had apparently concluded that I was overreacting to the pressures of motherhood, that I needed to calm down and I was fine to go home. At that I fled the room in tears, leaving Nick behind.

Go home? Me? I can't. I can't. I stumbled down the corridor, ran through the dining room and lounge and headed for my bed, sobbing hysterically. My mind was in complete panic and turmoil. I felt I was drowning. I could not breathe. I felt battered by all the drugs of previous weeks and now I was being thrown out of the environment that I was beginning to feel safe in. Visions of my last night at home, cutting my legs, haunted me. I remembered shaking Dominic and yet they wanted me to leave here? I'd hurt me. I'd hurt him. I did not want to but I just knew I would. In the midst of this panic and turmoil a sudden bolt came to me with no logic. I sat upright, sniffed and wiped my eyes, and with a surge of energetic defiance I thought, 'Blow them all! Obviously if they think there is nothing wrong with me and that I'm just wasting everyone's time then I must be. I've made all this up. I'm just copying the pupils I've seen in special schools. Right. Fine. I'll go then.' At that I frantically began throwing all my possessions into carrier bags, declaring loudly to a concerned patient, 'There's nothing wrong with me. I'm going home!'

Meanwhile, in the case conference, Nick had been having his say. He declared how unprofessional the situation had been, in that I had not been told it was to be a case conference in the first place; that none of these people had even been introduced to us; that all that had happened to me was a series of medication changes, none of which had really had a stabilising effect as yet; that he too felt that I was not yet ready to come home and asked what had happened to the original plans for gradual discharge. Surely, after almost three weeks, I should not just be sent home? Apparently the other professionals shifted uncomfortably and looked guilty. The social worker I had recognised spoke up and said that as she had known me prior to my current state then she felt justified to support Nick's belief that I was still far from well. She knew me as an intelligent, confident and efficient person, not the wreck they saw today. She fully recognised that I was sick, that I needed help and should not be sent home until I was ready. Nick then came to find me.

He and my named nurse met me in the corridor with my clothes spilling out over the top of a Tesco bag, shouting, 'Come on, I'm going home.' I headed for the side door out to the car park but Nick blocked my way. I fought with him, stating that we might as well go because there was nothing wrong with me. The nurse said it was my choice to go but she too did not recommend it. Nick was trying to encourage me to stay. Between them they calmed me down a little and the nurse told me that there were other things they could try for me. If I left now they could not help. She said either way I would have to go back briefly to the office to sign papers for my discharge. I followed her, clinging to Nick. In the office I sat feeling numb and quiet. The nurse said she would return to the others to enquire if any further decisions had been made. I knew I needed and wanted help. I wanted rescuing and Nick and I could not do it alone, so I was prepared to listen.

She returned a few minutes later and reported that the team had decided to continue my need to stay in hospital for the time being but with additional services and the suggestion to try electroconvulsive therapy (ECT) with me. The nurse explained that although some people felt it was an outdated method, it had worked for certain people like me and it might help. She gave us a leaflet to read with references from 1991. It looked old-fashioned and did not dispel the idea of it being an antiquated type treatment. The leaflet explained that it was a safe method which had been used for over 50 years and was effective. At my hospital it was carried out on two mornings per week. Prior to the first treatment I would have to have blood tests, a chest X-ray and a physical examination to check if I was fit enough, physically, to have the general anaesthetic, by injection. It outlined a number of rules which must be adhered to, such as wearing flat shoes and loose-fitting clothes. It warned of a headache following treatment, and that a nurse from the ward would accompany me. The information went on to state that it was not an immediate cure but may take several treatments before any benefits showed, although one side-effect could be some memory loss. The number of treatments given would be determined by the doctor in charge of my case. I still pictured, in my mind's eye, a scene from a black and white film, with a patient tied down to a bed, jumping around as electrodes were applied, before going back to their ward in the 'loony bin'!

Nick and I were left to think it over. I was desperate for something to work and decided, in spite of my mental images, to try it. I unpacked my bags, washed my face and settled down to wait again for the next drinks trolley and lunchtime, feeling confident that something was going to help me. Later on that day Nick took me to my parents' house for a brief visit as Dominic was there. I did not stay long but at least it was a little progress.

After the outcome of the big case conference, Nick was able to see our GP who signed him off work for several weeks to cope with his current demands. At school they decided to disband his class and share the assistants out to assist with the problems caused by poor supply cover in my area. The Hanzaks were not popular but this was the least of our worries.

My ECT treatment could not take place until I had been given the appropriate physical tests. Nick had to take me to the general hospital for some of them, including a CT (computed tomography) scan. I felt very claustrophobic as I lay on the table, as the large machine was passed over me, but the whole appointment was a terrifying ordeal. I was now very, very nervous at unfamiliar places and panicked if other people were too close to me. I did manage another trip to my parents for a 'goodbye' meal with my brother and his family. Although I did not feel it at the time, in retrospect I felt guilty for ruining that family Christmas and their stay with us in England. My illness caused problems for many people and this included them.

I went home to take the Christmas decorations down. I remember feeling a little sad that Dominic's first Christmas had not been one anyone had wished for, but certainly did not dwell upon it as I still felt detached from him. As he played with the beads from the tree, we took a photograph of him. His face looked blotchy but he was sitting up, wearing a bright blue Arran cardigan I had made. He was losing the real 'baby' stages but I was oblivious to it. Claire said he had begun to look like the character Grant Mitchell from the television soap opera *Eastenders*! I remember feeling extremely low, back on the ward, after this visit. I would have appreciated a chat with a nurse but there seemed to be none available. An opportunity should be made for patients, like myself, to be given a debriefing session after a visit home and chance to air their successes or concerns. This would be a valuable tool to aid recovery. I felt, at this point, that as a mother all my duties were delegated. I did not feed Dominic, change him, choose his clothes, bathe or put him to bed. Even Cathy took him to be weighed and checked at the clinic. They suggested even more creams for his skin. With hindsight, I wonder if the deterioration in his skin was due to the sudden withdrawal of my milk. One reason I had persevered with breast-feeding was that it was supposed to help eczema. Yet again, though, I did not give this a second thought at the time as I was just glad to be free.

One big improvement that Dominic had made was that he now slept through most nights for his father. Although naturally I was pleased that Nick was at least able to sleep better, I was so self-centred, I did not really care either way. It actually just made me feel even more distant from my child because it made it clear to me that it was obviously all my fault Dominic did not sleep. I was a useless mother anyway, so other people might as well take him over. They did a better job.

A week or so after the awful case conference I went for my first ECT treatment. There were four of us from the ward who were escorted across the lawned area outside our ward to a smaller building. A nurse took us and we waited in a room which resembled a café, with red plastic chairs and a drinks area. There were a couple of groups similar to ours and a few others who must have been outpatients. I was nervous but saw some other patients called into another room. A few minutes later they would return with a slightly glazed look and pink cheeks. They were given a drink and then escorted back to where they had come from.

Soon it was my turn. I was taken into a bright room with a bed in the centre. There were four staff members standing by it. One asked me to sit on the bed and remove my shoes. I lay back on the white sheets and thought how comfortable the bed was. A doctor took my arm, rolled up my sleeve and told me there was nothing to worry about. He told me I would feel a scratch and should count out loud. I felt the tingle of anaesthetic climb up my arm and only got to five. In those moments I felt the best peace since 'floating' on morphine when I was pregnant. I understood why drug addicts seek solace in their addiction. Imagine you have had a very busy day or long journey when all you can think of is getting into bed. Eventually you find yourself between the sheets, snuggle down and begin to drift into the twilight period of falling asleep. That feeling had evaded me for so long and now at last I could experience it again. This was what I needed – my brain switching off. I could have been unconscious for hours, I did not know. Initially I became aware of someone saying my name and gently tapping me. Consciousness returned as I focused on four faces smiling at me, asking if I was all right. Gradually I sat up and realised I had a headache like that of a hangover. My shoes were passed back to me and slowly a nurse guided me back to the café area. Then I realised my 'trip' had been a matter of minutes as I had glanced at a clock prior to my treatment. I was given a drink of tea and sipped it. My teeth felt sensitive, as if I had accidentally bitten on the foil from a biscuit wrapper. We returned to the ward and were encouraged to have a rest to 'sleep it off'. After my first treatment, the headache continued for a few hours. I was very tearful that evening and the next day my whole body ached. I was concerned that if I felt so battered by the treatment, then some of the fragile, elderly ladies who also were given ECT must have felt even worse. With each subsequent treatment, however, these side-effects lessened, and an hour or so after the treatment it felt like nothing had happened to me.

I continued to have visits home more regularly the next week. Some were successful, with me doing a couple of basic chores and just playing with Dominic. On others I would feel like a stranger in my own home, uncomfortable and feeling frightened. I always looked forward to going back to the ward and missed it when I was absent. The visits were increasing until one Sunday afternoon I came home and panicked about everything so much that Nick basically took me straight back. The pressure of loading the washing machine and making a drink proved too much and I caved in. Back in hospital I hurt myself again, intentionally, and had a very bleak evening, tearful and restless. Another down point and I did not go home again for eight days. The doctor had 'grounded' me.

In the meantime, they had suggested another couple of activities for me in the hospital. I had a few appointments with a physiotherapist who went through some simple relaxation techniques. The first time I was due to see her she came to the ward to collect me. She was a friendly, middle-aged lady who I warmed to within seconds. She took me down some of the long corridors to her department. We went into a small, dimly lit room which had beanbag chairs, a comfortable chair plus a padded, adjustable couch. I was to lie on that and make myself comfortable. I did not stop talking initially! She was the first person for weeks I felt I could chat to and I poured it all out. However, this was not part of the treatment she was to give me and tactfully tried to tell me so. Slightly disappointed, I went quiet as she began to make me think of the different parts of my body. Twitch. Twitch. Fidget. Giggle. It did not work at first. She then made me visualise a candle. I could do that one all right. I then had to breathe on the imaginary candle just enough to make it flicker but not go out. I did it. I cried. Big sobs. It had reminded me of birthday candles. I love birthdays. Happy times. I wanted to be happy but I did not know how to be any more. She let me cry silent tears and passed me a tissue. Whilst I lay there she began just to chat to me about how this department was closing in a couple of weeks. She told me her holiday plans and then of her new post on her return. I listened. Then we went back to thinking of a candle. I breathed slow and calm breaths. I began to relax a little.

She walked me halfway back to my ward and let me return alone. I felt much calmer and looked forward to my next sessions with her. Due to the closure I only managed a few but each time the techniques became easier. She also tried some acupuncture on me. I was intrigued, but I do not know if it had any real effect upon me. I was so proud of myself the first time I walked to and from her department myself. Prior to my illness, I had considered relaxation to be easy enough. I would find some household chores relaxing; tinkering jobs in the study; some television programmes and knitting. All of these had begun to elude me. I have never really been a person who can relax by 'just sitting', but this was what I now had to learn to do. At least with the daily mundane pressures taken off me I could concentrate just on me. For those weeks in hospital I really appreciated all the meals and drinks being sorted for me. The only decision I had to make was at the serving hatch as to my choice of cooked meal. The routines gave you security, yet if you wanted to you could set the tables and be a little more involved. As my symptoms had worsened at home in December and I broke down under the strains of my life, the task now was to rebuild every aspect in ways I could manage. My mind had become so hyperactive that initially the concept of concentrating just on breathing was impossible. With just a few of these relaxation sessions I had made another step in the right direction. I learnt that when my mind had been relaxed and cleared for a while then I was ready to take on a challenge.

Meanwhile I still was reluctant to go home again, even though I was improving within the security of the hospital. I was happy to see Nick and Dominic and we had several walks around the vast grounds. Nick would recall many of his childhood memories and I loved to listen to them. Unfortunately that week Dominic developed a cough and a sickness bug, so the sleep pattern went and so did his pleasant mood. He was grumpy and difficult. I was indifferent about it. Nick was exhausted. By the weekend my parents had Dominic for a couple of nights to help Nick, who also had begun a cold!

The next week I did begin to venture out to other places. Drinks at my mother-in-law's were a regular occurrence which I liked, but now we progressed to meals. Nick made a comment in Dominic's diary that I was getting much better. We had a big step forward as I suddenly announced I wanted to go to Marks and Spencer, buy some tasty food and take it home to cook and eat! In the car park I was very close to backing out of the idea but Nick said he would not leave my side. Every nerve in my body was on edge. I was so aware of the sounds – tills, voices, children. The lights seemed so bright. The shelves looked so big and the products so bright. Yet it was the people that really scared me. If anyone crossed my path I stopped dead as if I had been hit. I was not at all happy and clung to the hand I was holding. We then met one of the staff from school – oh no! What would they think about both of us 'off sick' yet we were well enough to be wandering around M & S! She said the classic comments, which still made me want to run and hide, 'Oh you look so well. I can't believe you've been in *that* hospital. Just think, too, you've got everything you ever wanted.'

I felt like I had been stabbed. Luckily Nick knew to make a hasty retreat and we headed quickly for the food. Then we met one of the mothers from my antenatal group. Utter panic! She chatted on to me about their Christmas and asked about ours. Oh dear – what could I say? I now felt embarrassed, awkward and ashamed when I told her where I had been. I blurted out that I was still 'in there' and this was my first trip to a shop. Her reaction was the best I could have wished for as she said how sorry she was and hoped I would soon be better. Amazingly, she offered immediately to visit me in hospital as she said she was quite used to going there as her own father had been in several times! I wanted to hug her with the relief. She suggested that she would arrange with Nick the best times to go and offered help in any way she could. Little did she know she had just prevented me having a crisis by the vase display! Encouraged by a true friend, who did then come to see me regularly, I managed to choose and make a meal back at home. Later on, Sue took me back to give Nick a rest and save him the journey yet again. Friends really can help with these small words and deeds and we both really appreciated them.

Next day I was feeling very brave and demanded another trip out – this time to IKEA, the furniture store. I was determined to handle it and all I wanted to do was walk through. Yet again my senses were on red alert. It was amazing how bright everything was. Displays seemed to be in 3D, and as if the colour button on a television had been turned up. Likewise, the whole store seemed very noisy. I was so sensitive to the proximity of other customers and wafts of perfume or body odours almost choked me. The only touch I was conscious of was Nick's hand in mine. I could feel my heart pounding in my chest. We wandered though the large room displays with me saying to myself, 'You're okay, you're okay, soon out.' Nick meanwhile was telling me the same thing. We went to the downstairs marketplace where they sell all the small items. Kitchen. Thump, thump of my heart. Pictures and frames. Thump, thump. Curtains and fabrics. Thump, thump. Bathroom. Thump, thump. Lighting. Thump, thump, thump, thump – sheer and utter panic. I do not know why but the effect of the lights above, beside and around me sent me into an utter terror, as if someone said a gunman was on the loose. I felt I could not breathe; there was no air, just lights, lights and people. I let go of Nick's hand and ran through the vast warehouse, desperate for escape. There seemed to be queues at all the tills and I could see no way out. Inside I was screaming with pure terror. Somehow I managed to find a way through. Nick found me outside, crying on a bollard.

'Take me back,' I said.

Next day I felt better but decided that just having a meal at home was enough. We both collected Dominic from Cathy's, who gave us the great news that his first tooth had appeared! At a later date Cathy told me she had really worried about telling me this, as maybe I should have discovered it myself – she certainly did not want to upset me or make me feel inadequate. Her kind concern was not necessary as I happily accepted the news. I actually fed, bathed, gave him supper and put him to bed that night before someone took me back to hospital. Nick commented in the diary on Dominic's behalf, 'I love my Mum.' It was just a pity that I still could not reciprocate it at this stage, but I was improving. After I successfully made a meal for our family at home, Nick took a photograph of Dominic and I having a cuddle in the spare room. We both look happy!

So Dominic's ninth month ended a bit better than the previous one. He had gained both in weight and length, in addition to his first tooth. He had not been to the doctor's once! He loved being in his door bouncer, baby walker and in the rucksack on his father's back. His favourite toy was Duplo shapes and he could clap his hands and stand supported. His heroic father had managed to get him to sleep through! He spent his nights at home but his days between his father and grandmothers and two days with Cathy. He visited me in hospital too. Overall he was doing well in spite of the dramatic changes to home life. I too was beginning to improve – maybe we would be a happy family one day.

CHAPTER 16

Looking up and outwards

Towards the end of January I was having regular ECT sessions. As the weeks went by my sleep pattern did begin to improve slightly. Initially I was only managing two or three hours' sleep spasmodically. I would lie awake just listening to the sounds of fellow patients sleeping. I would wave at staff as they did the occasional round, shining torches on us, but they just told me to go to sleep (I wish!). I was very, very lonely during those hours, often crying and rocking myself for comfort. This particular ward policy did not encourage patients to be up in the night as I had discovered. In reality, those hours were the worst of my whole stay. Many times I had to fight the urge to hurt myself but as the logical, balanced side of my brain began to work again these urges subsided. Usually by 4 a.m. I might have gone to sleep and then I would be woken up at 6.30 a.m. for a cup of tea, an hour and a half before breakfast time. Several times I just muttered 'no thanks' but was told off for being lazy! How I wanted to yell at them, 'Don't you realise how vital sleep is to me – I've hardly been able to sleep for months and you're waking me up telling me I have to come and have a revolting cup of tea?'

I suppose that was true hospital institutionalisation but I do not think a bit of flexibility would have hurt.

Gradually, with the combination of the relaxation techniques I had been shown, plus the effects of medication and ECT, at last I began to drift off to sleep much sooner. One feeling I would try to create was the thought of the anaesthetic working and imagine that luxurious sinking feeling. With improved sleep, of maybe five hours instead of two or three, I did begin to perk up in general. On the ward I started to enjoy watching television – always on loudly due to the deaf elderly ladies! I also started to spend hours doing jigsaw puzzles. This was a pleasure I had not had time to indulge in for years. One big improvement was my renewed interest in knitting. I did not want to do anything for Dominic at first but made some dolls clothes for friends' children. This led to a friendship of sorts with another patient. She too was a young mother but suffered from alcoholism. She had a little girl who loved dolls but she could not knit for her. I taught her and we spent many hours with pink frocks and blue coats! Eventually I did make a couple of items for Dominic, which was another step in the right direction.

I lost all interest in my appearance in hospital. My hair was long but neither curly nor straight. I just washed it and dried it without the usual fuss I make. I was told to keep my nails short but never painted them. All I wore were leggings and t-shirts. If I left hospital I always wore the same checked shirt. I looked forward to wearing my nightie and dressing gown each evening. My feet were permanently in a pair of blue fleece 'booties' with a pink collar! Make-up never touched my face. I was clean but that was all.

Another activity they recommended for me after another week was to use the hospital gym. It was a very old prefabricated building in the grounds. It was smelly and damp and only had a handful of antiquated exercise machines in it, but I liked it! A couple of young instructors were there to help you. They devised and went through simple fitness programmes with you. Little by little my performance improved and I began to feel the occasional adrenaline buzz. It felt good and reminded me of very happy days when Nick and I first became friends and we would spend hours in the gym keeping fit. Being reminded of good times sometimes motivated me to want to make them possible again. We had bought a child seat for Dominic to put on Nick's bicycle so we could exercise together one day soon.

Another step forward was my increasing use of the ward telephone. At first I would not speak to anyone and staff would just mention that my mother, for example, had rung to see how I was. My dependence on and love for Nick was very strong and increased the better I got. As my confidence improved I would occasionally say I would speak to him when he rang if someone else had visited me. His peace at home in the evening was shattered when I began to phone him! It is amazing how you can chatter on about nothing when you are 'in love'! The very fact that I had begun to miss him and started asking how Dominic had settled to bed was also a good sign. At home I would not answer the telephone but wait for Nick to deal with it.

In late January we all decided I should try to sleep at home for a night. It was strange for us all but I managed well. I even wrote in Dominic's diary for the first time in weeks. Nick took a morning photograph of 'mum and son' – again we both look very happy!

During these weeks I was still having ECT. One side-effect I had was that I definitely suffered from memory loss. Even when I read of the family events and activities that I was involved with at this time I have no recall of them whatsoever, even if given further reminders or clues. I apparently went out for meals with the family; to a large John Lewis shop; to see a show with my parents; for walks in local beauty spots and to see a film. Apparently we went out for a meal on Valentine's night with Sue and Jon! It is all lies as far as I am concerned – I was not there! From reading my comments in the diary, I obviously began to do more with Dominic and take pleasure in it. For example, I had a bath with him and noted that it was the first time he had lifted his arms to me when I said he had to get out. Social services were involved with us quite heavily and would call in frequently when they knew we would be at home.

My parents became more involved as my time out of hospital increased – probably due to me being more willing to see them too. We began spending weekends with them and my mother always made a roast dinner each Sunday for the family. This meant I saw my grandparents too, whom I had not been seeing. I knew my grandmother would be devastated to see me in hospital so I preferred to see her at home. I was slightly aware that people were concerned about me but I could not bear to see it. My grandmother is not good at hiding her worries and consequently she would have made me uneasy.

I continued to spend nights at home but Nick tended to see to Dominic if needed. It was a big step one morning when I wanted to get him up, give him breakfast and get him ready for the day. I think Nick must have been wary of my 'big ideas' as I was still volatile at times and what seemed a good idea one minute was terrible the next. Overall, though, I was improving with my desire and ability to meet his needs again and be less bothered by his inevitable cries. By this stage I had been an inpatient for around eight weeks.

However, I was still having many worries and I must have been encouraged to write down some of my thoughts, and Nick helped me. The idea was to recognise the positive and negative feelings I had and to identify some aims. These were my main thoughts around early February.

- I can't get thoughts, feelings and reactions into any form of true proportion, in relation to their actual importance, i.e. I feel that I'm either over- or under-reacting to nearly all situations and dealings with people.
- Although still knowing I have to return to work, I feel very angry and resentful at having to return and have the same feelings towards the changes that I know have taken place in my absence.
- I do not feel that I am the Elaine that I want to be (that I used to be in August).
- A circumstance that has changed is that Nick is now capable and confident at seeing to Dominic's needs (actually this is very good), but at the moment it makes me feel even more inadequate. I feel guilty and robbed of breast-feeding.
- I don't feel that so far during my illness that anyone, i.e. doctors, nurses, have given me any clear idea of the structure of how my condition runs. Decisions have been made and not clearly communicated back to me.
- I am normally an intelligent and perceptive person and do not feel that I have been treated as such.

- I still feel a strong urge to retreat from the pressures of everyday life, i.e. back to hospital.
- I still have a very strong desire to hurt myself, especially if I am disappointed over anything.
- Normally I do definitely have peaks and troughs in my emotional state but usually manage to maintain a more level approach to situations. At present the peaks and troughs are even more extreme and I cannot keep any form of level approach.
- Dominic was much wanted and planned but he has proved to be our greatest cause of problems – illnesses, pregnancy, time off work, sleeplessness, financial, time, change of lifestyle.
- I feel that all members of my family have been supportive.
- Generally I am lethargic yet I still have problems getting to sleep. I am tense and short tempered – like bad premenstrual tension.

I identified some possible 'spanners' to the family life I had imagined:

- being ill when pregnant
- traumatic birth
- problems with coping as a working mother
- childcare arrangements
- pressure to have a second child, like my peers have
- sleepless nights
- Dominic's illness
- trying to take on too much
- Dominic's endless minor ailments
- trying to please husband – high expectations not met
- onset of PND – change in drugs – no sleep.

I expressed my current concerns as:

- sleeping pattern is not good
- memory – getting better and I do not feel I am as gormless
- highs and lows – not as many, more even tempered, but still having lows for no apparent reason
- Dominic's 'bad spells'
- Nick going back to work.

From all this Nick and I tried to set a few aims, with the effects a week or two later in brackets:

- not to feel too bad about the end of breast-feeding *(getting better)*
- the more I do with Dominic, the closer I'll become *(happening)*
- maintain a positive attitude to returning to work *(abandon for the moment)*

- possible return to work part time *(abandon for the moment)*
- continue to make social arrangements *(done so but still worry and don't want to talk or return calls)*
- get some exercise *(yes! walk and swim)*
- try to get on with some normality *(Nick still around; housework and some shopping okay)*.

The inevitable change did happen when Nick returned to work after the February half-term. I was still not fully out of hospital but as he had to go back my mother took the next half-term off to support me. If I was at home for the night, Nick would take Dominic to her house on his way to school. This gave me time on my own to sleep or just potter around. Later in the day she would bring him back and the three of us would maybe go out for lunch or shopping. Initially I did not want to drive. It was another everyday task that now terrified me. The dreadful thought could suddenly cross through my mind when I did drive that I could hit another car or crash into a tree and part of me wanted to. Until thoughts like that subsided I was not safe at the wheel. Likewise, I could have a panic attack, like the one I had experienced in IKEA, if I was caught between two trucks. Just as with other tasks, I had to take it slow and steady, gradually building up again. The more places we went to, the more my confidence began to improve and my desire to drive began to return.

In addition to home visits by social workers and my health visitor, one regular person who became involved at this point was my community psychiatric nurse (CPN). He had been at the big case conference about me but his involvement was only due to begin when I was discharged. I liked him and began to look forward to his visits. He did not judge me but listened and made sensible suggestions. The first time he came to see me at home was my first morning alone with Dominic (I wonder if that was planned?). I was nervous about the whole morning but managed to survive. To celebrate, in the afternoon I tidied a big cupboard out at my mother's house!

By the end of Nick's first week back at work Dominic had a bad cold again and was not sleeping! My parents stepped in and gave us two nights without him. Everyone was on alert now not to let me slide in any way. At the hospital I had been moved from the main bedroom into a side room with only six beds in it. This was for the part-timers, as I had now become. The ECT treatment had stopped and I had begun to want to spend most of my time now at home. The need for the ward and its routines had reduced dramatically, as I was now able to manage at home with family support.

All three of us were invited to a case conference about Dominic held at a local clinic. Both Nick and I have been involved with such meetings on a professional basis but it felt very different to be 'on the other side'. The room seemed cold and dark as no one put the lights on. We sat in a circle on low, high-backed chairs around a small coffee table. I immediately felt threatened by everyone having papers and reports on their laps, some were clicking pens. I wanted to shout that we were real people, not bits of paper. Why should they need papers if they knew us well enough? If they did not know enough about us then why should they be there? For a person like me who has been buried in paper at work and home (diaries!) for years, it seems strange that I reacted this way. I did feel it put up a barrier immediately and that we were yet another case to be filed. There was a social worker, our health visitor, plus two community support workers, yet I felt there were more than four people. Apologies were sent from my psychiatric nurse, a family support member and the child protection officer. I am glad there were only the four. Everyone was pleasant but the basic concern was that without support, Dominic could be at risk from me. I know that was true but talking about it in such a formal way made me feel worse at a time when I was beginning to improve. Without the Christmas day incident this would not have happened. I do not blame Nick for reporting it but I do not think my involvement in this was productive towards my recovery.

The outcome of the meeting was to undertake a four-week assessment period to monitor my parenting of Dominic. So, just as I was beginning to get better I was on trial! The desired outcome would be that he would be safe in my care and that social services could withdraw. Tasks and responsibilities were drawn up, mainly for me to have visits by a series of different people. I agreed because I did not really have any option but the whole experience made me nervous, edgy and uncomfortable. I still felt I could put on an act to a certain extent. If my family could not see through that, then what good could these people do? No one had saved me from the fall into hospital so my faith in the system was not great either. After the meeting the three of us had lunch out. I had no appetite. Next day, however, my mother took Dominic and I for lunch in Cheadle – I ate plenty and felt good!

Around the same time I dictated to Nick my current feelings:

- I feel better generally about Dominic. I have been left alone with him briefly and taken him out by myself.
- Still feel robbed of breast-feeding; giving him a bottle just does not feel the same. It makes me feel that I have lost 'ownership' of him.
- I have made a few social arrangements and am looking forward to going away at Easter.
- I have driven the car!
- Enjoyed preparing some meals/cooking.
- Been out to cinema (Saturday).
- Been out for lunch (Sunday).
- My memory loss has caused me to feel a bit stupid on a number of occasions.

- I find it difficult to carry on conversations without losing my thread. I cannot seem to think of appropriate words to ask even in simple conversations. I feel that I am drifting off, going distant, feeling blank and numb towards everything.
- I still have great difficulty in getting to sleep.
- Generally feel more relaxed about all aspects of Dominic. No longer anxious about Nick's response to Dominic.
- Very worried still about taking on the pressures of everyday life. I find this very frightening.
- I feel I have generally behaved better this weekend, not felt as awkward towards people and situations, generally more relaxed.
- I feel that I am a bit closer to getting back to the Elaine that I like – but I am still some way off.
- I am still going to extremes of emotions – highs and lows.

Meanwhile by ten months our son was continuing to develop well. I was home most of the time and he had a busy time going out and about with his grandmother and me. He was responsive to most things and I began to enjoy hearing him chuckle in his door bouncer. He was almost 10 kg and 75 cm long. He preferred to sit rather than lie down and had developed a cute skill of getting on all fours and rocking back and forwards. He had learnt to shake his head and give us a cheeky look if told 'No'. Dom had taken an interest in the *Holiday* television programme and would smile and shout at Jill Dando, the presenter. He liked to play with his fingers on his lips and his party trick was to blow raspberries. He looked chubby!

CHAPTER 17

Discharge day!

By the end of February I was at home most of the time. I still had high and low moods with sudden drops or rises. I could be very lethargic and yawned a great deal. On bad days I had no enthusiasm, with blank or silly (self-harming) thoughts. On good days I was more even tempered and felt my sleep and memory were better. Generally everything seemed like a huge challenge, e.g. washing, ironing, choosing and preparing meals, which sometimes overwhelmed and frightened me. My negative fears and worries included driving, seeing friends, being alone and unable to do sewing/knitting at home as I found it hard to relax there. With Dominic I was better but still needed much support. Yet my dependency upon the hospital had actually reduced dramatically.

Consequently in late February I apparently attended my discharge meeting where my care programme was discussed and set, according to the paperwork I have, as I can not remember it. My care was to be passed from the nurse on the ward to my community psychiatric nurse (CPN) on discharge. Three main needs were identified. Firstly, practical support with Dominic was to be given by a representative from a family centre who would visit us twice a week. I had to aim to attend the well baby clinic at least once a month and contact my health visitor for advice, if needed at other times. Secondly, I was to be given emotional support and education of the effects of my illness and would have an assessment by a doctor from the Family and Psychotherapy Service. My CPN was to visit me weekly. Thirdly, I had to maintain my mental health by regular reviews of this and of my medication in outpatients. I was given a general leaflet about the 'Care Programme Approach'. This was a good idea and contained clear and simple information.

Nick came to collect me from the hospital on the final morning to bring me home for good (we hoped!). We probably both had mixed feelings of relief and happiness but also tinged with worry and concern for the challenges we still faced. Yet this had to be a happy day and I certainly was a healthier person than when I had been admitted ten weeks earlier. Back to being a family again with no more trips to hospital!

One suggestion from my CPN was to keep a diary about what I did from now on and how I had felt. Not only did I do Dominic's, I now had to write my own in a notebook. It had emergency numbers of the relevant nurses, social workers and family support people on the inside cover, who I could contact if need be. Initially my nurse would visit every few days and gradually lengthen the time between his visits. He would look at my diary and comment upon any issues which arose.

During the first few weeks at home I sometimes was disturbed by Dominic during the night. Both of us had a cold and cough which did not help. If I did not feel I could cope after a bad night, Nick would take Dominic to my mother's so I could go back to bed. Increasingly, I did manage myself and learnt to have a lazy day instead of rushing around after a bad night. Generally, though, I continued to be tired and lethargic. I often went back to bed after I had got Dominic ready to go to Cathy's. One day I went back to bed until 3 o'clock in the afternoon! I basically felt I had 'no get up and go' and this was my way of dealing with it. Occasionally I would feel very glad to send Dominic to Cathy's and would have a glum, bad tempered and cross day as a consequence. My guilt of palming my child off to someone else remained. After a string of disturbed nights again I took Dominic to the doctor's, mainly for reassurance. I was convinced by now that the disturbed nights were my fault, as why else did he sleep well when I was in hospital? The lovely male doctor gently suggested that it was probably due to him teething at present. I think he was just being kind to me, but nonetheless it gave me renewed strength to continue. If I had slept well I usually had a more productive and calm day than when I had been disturbed. I gradually began to convince myself that many chores simply did not have to be done when I felt they did. Why do the ironing today if it could wait until I felt better? If I overslept and missed going to a church coffee morning, for example, I learnt to tell myself that it did not matter. I began to play music again, often loudly, and would sing and dance around. This was excellent therapy. A few years later I spoke to a counsellor after three of my pupils died within a few months of each other. Amongst her good advice was to be kind to myself, 'appeal to your senses', she suggested. If anyone had seen me after that phone call they would have sent me back to hospital. There I was wearing my favourite dressing gown, sniffing my favourite aftershave Nick wears, eating chocolate, listening to a Lionel Richie track played loudly and looking at photographs which made me smile – all as I danced around the kitchen! It was wonderful therapy and I highly recommend it! Looking back, I had been on the right track. We often overlook our own needs in times of stress and grief, almost feeling guilty if we let ourselves go, even for a short time. Treating yourself like a best friend and allowing yourself pleasures is a strong tonic to help you cope with stressful periods.

The days when Dominic went to my mother or Cathy, I initially would retire back to bed or at least stay in my dressing gown until lunchtime. I would spend time over the post, my breakfast and the newspaper. I would do some of the basic household chores and choose easy meals to prepare out of the freezer. I continued to find therapy in tidying and sorting items, such as photographs. If Dominic and I were in ourselves we may go back to the big double bed and just play and read stories. Sometimes we both fell asleep again. At weekends Nick would bring me breakfast in bed – bliss!

I began to rekindle the warm bond between myself and my parents and grandparents, often having lunch at their homes or out in the community. I began to cope back amongst crowds, such as in Chester, around the shops. I was pleased when strangers complimented Dominic and if he smiled at them. Little by little my confidence to drive the car returned, although I still had to fight hard with myself to counteract the self-destructing thoughts I had behind the wheel. At least I could acknowledge now that they were just that, i.e. thoughts, and not actions. In a strange way, if these ideas arose I would get inner strength by pushing them aside and concentrating on the company or journey. I then could congratulate myself on an achievement. By the middle of March my mother had to go back to work again. I felt sorry but not too worried as I was beginning to cope much more. Gradually I managed going out alone or just with Dominic. One day I went to a garden centre and met neighbours of my parents plus other people I knew. I felt wary but realised that I would be embarrassed regardless of why I was 'off sick'. I definitely felt a stigma with my illness at this stage. I must have been feeling defensive too as I noted in my diary that 'at an NCT coffee morning I felt rather awkward but did talk to people about my hospital stay – no one said anything to upset me.'

As a family we began small outings at the weekends again. On my parents' wedding anniversary we had lunch out with them and had a walk along the Wirral Way. That evening my father showed us slides of days gone by. I found it good to look back at my childhood days as they were such happy memories. Probably a few weeks earlier it would have upset me and I would have cried, comparing this happy family with the one I did not feel I had. So this was progress! I complimented myself on several other achievements. For example, on a trip to my mother-in-law's I felt the most talkative there for months; I got dressed one morning before breakfast and felt bright; I went to see my next door neighbour for the first time in months; on a trip to John Lewis at Cheadle with my mother and grand-mother I drove the car, chatted to people in the Mother and Baby room and generally felt that I was in control; once I overslept for a doctor's appointment but coped with the rush. One day I wrote that I was 'chatty over tea. It's good to feel good! We decided to go away at the weekend.' All three of us joined my parents for a night's stay at the Copthorne hotel at Dudley again. I buzzed with excitement as I packed. We met up with Claire and my parents in the Merryhill shopping centre. However, I was more preoccupied with the people than the actual shops. Back at the hotel we had a family swim in the pool. It was a good feeling to watch Nick and Dominic together in the water. My stay in hospital had definitely made them closer. To save us all being potentially stressed eating in a restaurant, that evening we had a bedroom picnic and all relaxed! We were learning. The next morning I received my first Mothering Sunday card! I happily packed up; we shopped for food and came home. Nick's family joined us and I actually made a meal for eight people!

'Brilliant!! Feel good! 9.5 out of 10 sort of day,' I wrote.

I had many visits from the social services, as outlined in my care plan. On the whole I found their sessions quite comfortable and relaxed, although I maybe exaggerated my achievements in order to try to convince them I was better. Nick and I attended a social services conference about us at a family centre. I was not as bothered this time as there were only three professionals there, all of whom I was now quite familiar with. I was more able this time to recognise when I may need help, such as when Nick was due back to work after the Easter holiday, so they planned more visits for me that week. The support from my CPN was now to reduce to fortnightly instead of weekly, but the best progress was that social services would now withdraw unless the circumstances deteriorated again. Hurray! Nick then went back into work with one less worry! However, I did feel a little let down by one service. I received a letter from the Family and Psychotherapy Service stating that as I had not been in touch following their visit to me in February, when I said their support was probably not needed, that they would discharge me from the service if I did not contact them in the next 14 days. It made me feel like a debtor of some kind. It seemed too pointed and offended me at the time, whereas a phone call to check would have been appreciated instead. In retrospect a letter was a sensible policy, but my reaction illustrates that I still was not fully well.

I still had times when I was low. One evening Dominic was grumpy but it did not bother me, yet Nick talking about school did. I felt very ruffled and frustrated about my job, and still could not handle thinking or talking about it. Even a trip to the hairdresser's was a downer. My hairdresser was surprised about my recent 'adventures'. Normally I managed to put on a show for him. During this stage I just sat, quiet and glum, and still refused to have any length cut from my hair. I had this notion of wanting it to be long and flowing. I was tired and quiet at home too. Some days I just could not be bothered to make any effort. I had also begun to feel down about my weight, as I struggled to fit comfortably into spring clothes. At this point I did nothing about it. My GP suggested that it should be the least of my worries. One evening I went to the pictures to see *Jerry Maguire* with a friend. I had not seen her for months and felt quite uneasy in the cinema. I did enjoy the film and a chat but I felt I was loud and pushy. I did not like myself. Halfway home on the 20-minute drive in the darkness I had an awful panic attack. I felt like someone had suddenly emerged in the back seat and was about to stab me! I pulled over, turned the light on and checked the car to try to calm myself. Even though logically I knew it was safe, I was still *very* scared and tearful. I clung to the steering wheel, howling for Nick to come and rescue me. Eventually the sensible side of me began to kick in as I realised he could not leave Dominic, and what could we do with the car? Think candle. Think candle. My heart was still pounding but I knew I had to carry on. I put Lionel Richie on the cassette player and tried to sing loudly. At first all I could shout were words of encouragement to myself as I drove at less than 30 miles an hour, but little by little the music helped and at last I arrived home. I was as exhausted and drained as if I had just driven for six hours in torrential rain. I ran into Nick, sobbing.

'But you *did* it,' he said. 'You got yourself home – well done!'

My feelings for Dominic began to emerge more strongly. He had his photograph taken by a professional photographer with a stand in a supermarket. He behaved and posed impeccably and I felt proud of him! I was pleased to witness, and wrote in my diary, any developments he made, e.g. 'Dom made a few crawling movements across the room!' As part of my care plan I took him along to the baby clinic to be weighed. It was not a success as I felt very wary of all the other 'coping' mothers there and could not leave fast enough. If I took Dominic to see a GP, I was fine and felt confident and efficient – it was groups of people which still made me uneasy.

As the month progressed, so did I. Against Nick and my mother's advice, I resumed taking my grandparents shopping again. It was a challenge but made me feel proud when I succeeded. I also learnt to relax a little more in the evenings and began to knit again. Another big step I made was to actually answer and begin to use the telephone from time to time. If Nick was in I tended to let him deal with calls but just occasionally I would do so myself. One day I telephoned Sue. There was an obvious silence from the other end although she had answered and said 'hello'. After a few moments she warmly congratulated me on my achievement – for months she had been the one making all the calls, even if just to chat away on the answer phone, when she knew I was there, unable to pick it up. Hearing my voice when she answered had this time almost made her cry with relief at a sign of my recovery. Recently I had begun to at least converse on the phone but here I was initiating a call! I had not actually acknowledged this progress until she pointed it out.

My weight was still annoying me so I made an attempt at some exercise classes again. The first time I went it was very hard and made me irritable all day. Poor Nick was on the receiving end of this. He still had to tread carefully, on the whole. Dominic stayed the occasional night with my parents to give us some space together, but we still slept in separate rooms because I was so restless when asleep and continually disturbed him.

My belief from the assertive training course that 'if something is worrying you, do something if you can to solve it' began to be my focus.

One evening I became anxious about all the things I had to do in the house – most were probably unnecessary, but at the time were important to me. So I stayed up late and busied myself in the study, but at least I went to bed feeling calmer. Some days I recognised that I did not want to be alone so would call to see my mother at work, then go to Mums and Tots, for example. Yet I still would praise myself in my notes if I successfully coped with the people there, so it must have remained an ordeal! An added relief was the discovery that one of our savings plans would mature that June and help ease financial worries.

Towards the end of March I went to see my CPN at the day centre. It was the first time I had been to him and not vice versa. He had kept trying to convince me that my problems had been an illness, but at this point I wrote, 'I am not convinced, as I know it is because I have failed at so many things. He was pleased with me generally. I decided to stop worrying about work until I got home and Nick reminded me that I have to go back. I had an early night – feel ruffled and tired.'

The following day I explained to my GP my need to be 'in control' of my life and events. Maybe this was why I had become fanatical that everything in our house was tidy. After our chat I felt better and I made a spontaneous decision to take my sick note into school – a huge leap of progress! My heart was pounding the whole time but I managed normal conversations with the office staff and the head teacher, knowing that everyone else would be busy in their classrooms. I could not handle any more than this but at least I had actually gone into the building. From there I had lunch with my grandparents, then stayed chatting to people at Mums and Tots when I collected Dominic. From here both of us went to the baby clinic and I stayed talking with another mother from my antenatal group for the first time. Usually I rushed out from all the other perfect mothers and good babies with whom I felt I could not compete. Back at home I had a pleasant visit from a colleague, Larry, who works at another school. It had been a very busy and good day for achievements but I had found it all very hard work, felt nervous and unsure underneath in all the situations. I continued to get very flustered at events out of my control, for example when my father was delayed in picking me up for an occupational health appointment. When I got to the relevant building they were behind schedule too so I had the chance to calm down before I was seen. I explained my current state and was reassured there was no pressure to go back to work just yet. The county doctor was a lovely, smart lady who took time to listen and reassure me. I think if I was a malingerer she would detect it though! On the way home my father and I called at Sainsbury's where I met a mother from a school I had once worked at. She quizzed me on why I was not at work and I was stuck for half an hour talking to her. I did not have the confidence to be assertive enough to make my excuses and depart. I was exhausted by the time I got home and just sat down all evening.

Sue and Jon had asked me to be godmother for their daughter, Katie. I was delighted to accept but the night before her christening I was in a terrible mood. My panic about the service manifested itself into a major soul searching hour or two. I tormented myself about thoughts of work and annoyed myself about it. All I wanted to concentrate on was the present time and enjoying Dominic. I did not sleep well, in spite of my medication. Next morning, though, we were up early and were soon all organised for Katie's christening. I was pleased we all looked smart and we had a family photograph. I coped reasonably in the church but was very nervous and uneasy standing up at the font as godparent. Sue had said I did not have to go up to the front during the service but I felt I was not doing my duty properly if I stayed in my pew. As we stood around Katie, I focused on her all the time and did not look at the congregation at all. I felt very awkward during the coffee session afterwards in the church hall, even though it was the same venue as Mums and Tots. I did not feel I was very sociable back at Sue's house and made a hasty exit. I used to be such a sociable person who could chat to anyone – where had that person gone? Months later Sue told me that one of her astute guests had commented to her that there was 'something not quite right with Katie's godmother – it's in her eyes, they're sort of flat.'

Later on that day we packed up and headed south to an apartment in Warwickshire. My parents had already stayed there a few nights, but as it was small we could not all stay together. It had a double bedroom, pull-down sofa bed in the lounge and a kitchen/dining area. We all had a walk around the grounds and a meal together before my parents left us to it. We watched television and set up the travel cot for Dominic in the small inner hall area. I eventually began to relax by bedtime, but it had been a stressful day and I was exhausted. Being in a strange place, Dominic did not sleep well and was with me most of the night on the sofa bed. Next day we had a swim, a walk around Stratford-upon-Avon and made a meal back at the apartment, before a bike ride. I loved being on my bike. I loved the wind on my face and hair. I felt free and it always reminded me of when Nick and I went camping and cycling in Norfolk one idyllic, Whitsuntide holiday before we were married. There was a heatwave and we had cooked bacon for breakfast, ate wonderful pub lunches, had barbeques for tea and were passionate morning, noon and night! We cycled through lavender-filled fields and on perfect beaches. Those were the days! Yet today had also been good in different ways and it was great to feel no pressure at all.

Our remaining days at the apartment were spent busily in order to keep Dominic amused, but at a leisurely pace. I was pleased to be able to navigate us around unfamiliar areas, restoring one skill I had. Some tourist places were too busy and noisy for me so we tried to avoid them. The best tonics were the bike rides, for us all. One evening we went through a little ford three times because it made Dominic laugh. He looked very cute on the back of Nick's bike and was bundled up in a padded suit, gloves, hat and thick bootees. However, the strain and tiredness began to tell on Nick who became bad tempered as we strolled around Leamington Spa. I decided to take Dominic and give him some space for a while. By the time we met up for a drink we all felt better. I guess at the time I did not realise what a worry I was. It had only been a month since my discharge from hospital and, although I was improving, Nick must still have been wary and watching for any relapses in my recovery.

Hence Dominic's 11th month ended on a positive note. We were on a family holiday and, although tiring and a bit stressful, were basically enjoying it! Although his sleep pattern was yet again non-existent, he had learnt to crawl and stand up against furniture. He had some teeth and had developed a liking for chocolate, bread and ice cream. He had also learnt to say 'No'! Dominic loved outings and was interested, bright and alert wherever we took him. He was no longer on the 'at risk' register and had a mother who was taking greater pleasure at being with him again.

CHAPTER 18

He's almost one!

Our Easter holiday continued, and Claire joined us at the apartment for the final two nights – Dominic would not go to sleep! Consequently by early the next morning I felt very weepy. After a walk and a meal back at our apartment, we all relaxed and discovered that four big lumps had appeared on Dominic's gums. This gave me another excuse on which to blame his constant demands. Claire took a couple of photographs of the three of us. Nick looked glum and exhausted; I was pale, drawn and tired but smiling; Dominic was almost smiling but not impressed at having to sit still! The strain definitely showed and it was not a photograph for a frame.

The next week was pleasantly spent with all three of us at home. I had lie-ins and rests when I needed them and took a greater interest in cooking our meals again, often assisted by Nick. Dominic now had a travel cot/play pen in the dining room. He could at least play safely there and watch us whilst we were busy in the kitchen. If not, by now it would have been mayhem trying to keep him in one place. He was fast in his baby walker as well as crawling. When we originally looked for a house, one of my requests was for a through kitchen/dining room for such reasons. At least one of my decisions was right! During the week we also had some local bike rides and did some gardening and grocery shopping. One day we left Dominic with Nick's mother whilst we went to some bigger stores in search of a stair gate. Unfortunately I felt very nervous and panicky again – oh dear. A nap back at home revived me and that evening I had a drink and chat with Debbie in Stockton Heath. I drove home happily, singing along to the radio, and congratulated myself on the progress I had made since the cinema trip. No panics this time.

I saw my GP and described the continuing roller coaster I was on, but generally that I was beginning to have more good spells. When I was first discharged my CPN, and others, advised me that initially I would have the occasional 'happy time' during parts of a day. Gradually this would increase to longer periods, e.g. a morning or afternoon. Ultimately I would have whole days of feeling better, with just the odd relapse. At this stage I guess I was about halfway through this process. It was a good piece of advice and helped me to rationalise the bad times. Instead of dwelling upon them I tried to focus on when my spirits and abilities would lift again. My

GP suggested I now stopped taking sleeping pills but to continue with the same dosage of antidepressants.

I had a very good day when Nick's friends, Roy and Beverley came. We visited show houses at Northwich, then went to a craft centre and had a walk in Delamere Forest with them. When Dominic had gone to bed we had a fondue meal. This was easy to prepare and, hence, stress free for me. As I had stopped taking the sleeping tablets I had plenty of wine to drink, felt exceedingly mellow and danced for hours! It was the first time I had really let my hair down for months. Beverley and I put the stereo on loudly in the lounge, turned the lights down low and boogied for England, leaving the men putting the world to rights in the dining room. What a tonic! Next day I saw my CPN who was pleased with my progress, despite the hangover.

Towards the end of that week I took Dominic and my grandparents for an appointment at the general hospital. I was pleased with Dominic in the waiting room as he played so well with some other children for almost two hours until my grandfather was seen. We had lunch at Marks and Spencer where I asked to jump the queue due to a fractious child and two weak, almost 90-year-olds – what assertiveness! A week or two earlier and I would not have been as brave. Later my parents returned from a holiday and we made a spontaneous decision to have fondue for the night with them and Claire. Once again I coped well and enjoyed it.

Nick's final day before going back to work was spent in our usual busy manner. We left Dominic at my parents whilst we had a trip to a garden centre. Back at my parents later I had an urge to do their garden. I did so and we all stayed for a meal, before going home for a relaxed evening watching television. An hour after we had gone to bed, I went in the spare bed leaving Nick to sleep peacefully. I could not sleep as I had become extremely upset, worried and nervous. In my rising panic and over-whelming distress, I managed to find a little bit of sensible logic to overcome it. I decided to write it down.

Get rid of it – need sleep – can't sleep – too uptight.
Why?
Nick back to work tomorrow. I'll miss him; I don't want him to go but he has to. I'll be okay (I think) but I don't like it. I like him around and I feel stronger and more confident with him about. I can cope if he is with me. Mum and Dad are both at work tomorrow. Again more concerns on my own – enjoyed Mum off with me. No lady from social services – I'd anticipated tomorrow being tough and she's cancelled.

I JUST WANT TO BE ME AGAIN.

Church coffee morning – told them I'll go back for the first time and now I'm really worried about it ... People ... Chat ... Talking ... they know I've failed; been weak; loopy. What do I say? What do they say?

Sleep/tiredness – feeling exhausted again – fifth night on no sleeping tablet. Not as tired in the day but it takes a while to get to sleep then wake up myself or Dominic starts.

Feeling panic I can't cope about all the above. Horrid feeling again. Want to hide but want to climb out again. Mum said I've not to get tired and start it all again. Feeling like this started it and got more and more out of control. Get rid of worries – put them in a box for now ... carry on list.

Work – had been feeling fine that September is months away before I may start properly. Last two weeks flown by. Panic again that I can't cope by September – running to make progress and getting nowhere. What if I'm not? Money worries me too???

HOPEFULLY I WILL BE FINE.

People – fear of/no confidence.
Why?
Been ill – always takes adjustment.
Mental illness therefore confidence affected even more so.
Shame/embarrassment associated with illness – me and them.
Questions/pressure of conversation – find it very hard to be two-way and ask about them, but do not want to talk about me. Therefore Dominic is a good diversion – he'll be with me tomorrow. Don't like the phone – he's not there. It's just me – that's not enough yet. Feel small and insignificant.

I *can* cope on my own and it's easier, so why bother with others? I guess I need to be able to communicate again to work. Normally I like to be sociable. Dominic is better when we are busy.

Help lines
I'm in the spare room because I don't want to disturb Nick – not because I'm martyred.
Ring Mum – she'll come out of work. Bit drastic but not impossible. Could try to ring CPN for a 'you're doing well' chat.
Don't go to coffee morning – but more failure. Want to go as really it's another step up – probably be okay.
Don't worry – been on sleeping tablets for a few months – need to adjust again – may take a while. Don't push yourself. Calm down now, read a magazine – at least resting.

It's ME who has set 'plan'. Time will tell. Still got May, June, July, August and plenty of April. Think of New Year's Eve in hospital – three months ago and I'm much further on than then.

Positives
- Dominic – enjoy and cope with him – love?
- Driving – okay.
- Family – okay.
- Shopping – okay.
- Home life – okay – tea, washing, etc.

Cope better if I don't plan to go somewhere and have chance to worry, e.g. visit to school. Maybe I should do this for a week or two, i.e. go with the flow?

Positive things I have done
- Mums and Tots – been.
- Clinic – been.
- Both Sues, NCT – been.
- Seen Debbie, Roy and Beverley, Carol [previous neighbour].
- School – boss and office – been.

To do
- Attend own church coffee morning.
- Jeannie – waiting to phone.
- Swimming.
- School – rest of staff.
- Make phone calls.

Action plan
If I don't want to go to my church tomorrow – I won't.
Write to Jeannie and explain about the phone, i.e. I don't like to use one.
Keep remembering all the good things I've done and improvements – look how logically you've done this with no silly thoughts about knives, etc.
Food and exercise – felt better for losing 4 lb and getting into clothes – slipped due to Easter. Be good again from tomorrow.
Enjoyed doing Mum and Dad's garden today – go back and do more.
Make hair appointment.

BE NICE TO MYSELF.
NO pressure to do anything.
ENJOY MYSELF.

I put the pen down and went to sleep. After this manic self-counselling I did actually sleep well and after Nick went back to work next morning, Dominic and I had a happy bath together. I had, and continue, to regret not feeling his bare skin against mine as soon as he was born, as this had been a sensory experience I had dreamed of for so long. Small pleasures, such as a bath together, did go a little way to compensate for this loss and strengthen my bonding with him. After this we actually went to our church coffee morning! I handled it reasonably well although I felt nervous for all the reasons I had identified the previous night. My positive mood continued most of the day and I even made a phone call to Jeannie – she was out! I resisted the urge to eat chocolate until late afternoon and made myself an appointment to have my hair done. I did some shopping for my mother and went to a one-year reunion of my antenatal class. Dominic kept hugging other babies and I felt very quiet. I still found it difficult to accept that all the other mothers seemed to have sailed through their child's first year, whereas I was continuing to struggle. I went home feeling a little subdued but did the ironing and made the tea. Dominic was crotchety too but I coped with him. By the end of this day I was tired (I am not surprised, in retrospect), but still felt like I was trying to go uphill all the time. Looking back I can now recognise that I tried to fit far too many things into a single day. I suppose I had been trying to prove to everyone, including myself, that I could manage everything. I thrive on being a busy person but probably made matters worse by still trying to do so much. I felt guilty if I sat with a drink, whilst Dominic played or slept. Silly me. My family continued to try to discourage me from the hectic schedule I planned for myself, but I took no notice.

Over the next few weeks Dominic's sleeping pattern continued to be varied, and so was mine. Most nights he slept through, and if he did wake it was briefly at around 4 a.m. One night he disturbed because his bottle had leaked water so the cot bedding needed changing. Other early mornings I would wake confusing the dawn chorus for Dominic crying. I would get up to see to him and then realise it was a false alarm. Our morning routines were pleasant in that Nick would change and bring Dominic into me when he got up for work. Dominic and I would play games until he had gone, then have breakfast and get ready for the day, occasionally having an extra nap. I began to admit, in my diary, that I was enjoying my cuddly times with him. We developed our routines, for example he would sit on my dressing table, exploring interesting items, whilst I put my make-up on. I had begun to take pride again in my appearance, which was a sign of recovery too. Most mornings when Dominic went to Cathy's I would treat myself to a lazy morning in bed. I was beginning to learn a little more about being kind to myself, in this way. These sessions gave me the energy to continue to be busy when I had my son all day.

Our days were spent with our busy schedule, including swimming; Mums and Tots, where I felt much better talking to people some days; visiting both Sues, one of our favourite pastimes; NCT coffee mornings, where I would feel a bit awkward initially but relaxed and chatted for a while if Dominic was good; shopping in a variety of stores and seeing my grandparents. As the month progressed I resumed more adventurous outings with my grandparents and Dominic to garden centres, hospital appointments and shopping. On one trip we got stuck in a traffic jam but I survived the stress. Another day my mother and I went to John Lewis at Cheadle for Dominic's birthday presents. We had no luck so went on to Chester instead! A big, round trip of almost 90 miles and I drove! These days I would not even contemplate this in one day.

I did, however, learn some ways to give myself a rest at other times, e.g. if Dominic was asleep in the car when we got home after a trip, I would put the car into our garage so I could rest myself without worrying (the garage side door opens directly into the kitchen so I could hear when he awoke). If Nick went out for the occasional evening, I relaxed by having a beauty session myself. Unfortunately I had had my hair permed but it still was not really how I wanted it. It was just wavy and hung there! Poor Richard must have dismayed at me ignoring all his advice to keep it straight! I continued to find helping my parents, and others, to be therapeutic for me. If someone was upset and I managed to console them it would give me a buzz that I was still of use. I particularly liked to weed and tidy my parents' garden. As both were working it was too much for them, and I found it therapeutic, even though they said I should not be doing it. They also had a new kitchen fitted and I was pleased to be able to help out by cooking an evening meal for us all whilst it was being done.

I began to cope better with chores around our own home too. On a sunny and windy day I succeeded in washing, drying, ironing and putting away a huge amount of laundry, much to Nick's surprise, and mine! I also succeeded in going into school another day, on the spur of the moment. I chose to go when I knew the staff room would be full and also went up to see my class in the school bungalow. Dominic was passed around the staff in the playground too. It was a big step forward for me and I confessed to having enjoyed it, although it had been a challenge. Around this time I saw my GP and CPN who told me to stop doing my own 'thought' diary as he did not think I needed it anymore. So it was back just to doing Dominic's again and to concentrate on living our lives. I continued to have a constant round of appointments with professionals, but they were becoming less frequent.

There were times I found difficult; for example, one afternoon after Nick came home we all went to collect a cream prescription for Dominic. We waited 45 minutes and all got cross and bad tempered with each other. After an unsuccessful shopping trip to look at swings and buggies I felt illogically down for the rest of the day. Some evenings I felt inexplicably miserable and would try to analyse why. At times I still wanted to hide, was scared of most things and in a 'can't be bothered' mode. It was moods like this which made me realise that I still needed to take my antidepressant tablets, and taking them was a ritual I insisted on daily. If I had a lie-in I would initially panic that I was late in having them, thus losing some of the extra energy and calmness the rest had given me.

I did, however, take notice of some of the ways in which Dominic was developing, with increasing pride. For example, he pretended to use his toy phone when playing. He had his first crawl on the grass but looked very worried about the sensation on his hands and knees. He was much quicker climbing the stairs and liked to be chased. Dominic was now waving and trying to say 'bye bye' when appropriate. At the clinic the health visitor commented he was crawling, and alert and interested. She noted his improved sleep pattern and gave advice about vitamin drops.

One weekend, after establishing that we could get a loan, we dropped Dominic off at his grandparents and we went to chose ourselves a VW Golf car. Our current Maestro needed a great deal spending on it so it seemed better to trade it in. It was also a treat for Nick. He loves cars and such a project hopefully would give him a 'lift'. It was not easy at home or work for him. To ease his pressure they had made some internal changes and the classroom that he had been in for years had been restructured, and a new role created for him. There were continuing problems which my absence created. Every day he was still greeted by people asking how I was and he did not know what to say. If he said 'fine' then that implied I should be in school. I was still very up and down and must have been hard to cope with. His sleep was disturbed either by Dominic still or more usually now by me. Since the ECT treatment I had developed severe whole-body spasms as I drifted off to sleep which made Nick jump as if there was a problem I had heard. Sometimes I would be aware of it but not always. When I was asleep I would be almost 'running' with my legs and constantly give him sharp kicks. If I was still I might snore! Some nights I could not get to sleep so I would move beds rather than disturb him. Waking up in the same bed rarely happened.

On Dominic's first birthday I took a 'good morning' photograph of him standing up in his cot waiting for us, before taking him through to our room for more. Nick looked very unenthusiastic, looking at his son as if to say 'What a year!' I cannot blame him. It definitely had not been what we had planned and nothing like the idyllic 'Baby Care' project I wrote at school when I was 13. I had previously discovered this in our loft one day amongst my keepsakes and we had looked at it together. I had lovingly cut out and stuck a collage of beautiful, perfect babies on the front, back and inside covers. The largest photograph was of a child, not unlike Dominic, sucking its thumb! I had compiled the text from a selection of books and leaflets which my mother had been given when Claire was born. Looking back it was now very dated advice, e.g. 'Most mothers become so involved with the excitement, happiness and chores of caring for a new baby that they are in danger of not taking enough rest to be able to cope with the additional work and responsibilities. They may have to let some of the housework go rather than neglecting their husbands. They should discuss any problem with him and ask his advice. If there are any other children in the family, the parents should try and pay extra attention to them and share the new baby together and all take part in the pleasure and excitement.'

Did I really write that? At the time it was graded by the teacher as 'very good – a well thought out and thorough project'. Nick has always teased me about this project and says that my rosy perceptions of motherhood and family life were all based on it. I have to agree that he is right!

We helped Dominic unwrap a few presents and plenty of cards. He liked the ones with badges on. We got him the current chart CDs for his memory and keepsake box. He was not impressed at this point but liked eating the paper. We spent the afternoon at the home of one of our pupils for her 21st birthday. I coped quite well with the handful of school staff who were there and luckily Dominic was the model child. I still looked pale and drawn in photographs.

The following day was Dominic's main celebration as I invited all the family to our house for a party. We were all kept amused by his reactions to his many new toys, especially 'tooting' a trumpet and sitting on a plastic tricycle. I felt quite at ease. I had ordered a proper birthday cake for him and had to stop him from grabbing the big 'Number 1' candle. A happy birthday candle – at last! Nick helped him blow it out. I just made the flame flicker! Dominic was lovely the whole day, pleasant, happy and entertaining. Next day we had a 'leftovers' party for both Sues and their children.

My parents gave me another beautiful white Royal Worcester figurine of a mother and baby looking at each other. It is called 'First Smile'. They had also given me similar ones when he was born and on Mothering Sunday called 'First Love' and 'First Kiss', respectively. They are classic reproductions of how a mother is supposed to feel for her child. At last I was beginning to feel this way a little myself. I just wished that everything still could be easier. Life continued to be a struggle in every way, regardless of how it appeared to others.

On reflection, though, we now had a boy who was one. He virtually slept through most nights and had a few naps in the day. He liked to feed himself breadsticks and rice cakes; ate mashed food or baby meals, yoghurt and fruit and liked titbits from an adult's plate. His favourite foods were grapes and chewing melon rind! His 12th month had been healthy with no doctor visits and he now had four teeth, with others about to appear. He could crawl fast and move along furniture. He had a few sounds that resembled words and loved being tickled. He liked to tease, giving and taking things. His typical day was now a play with me in bed; going to a coffee morning; lunch out; shopping; visiting grandparents; evening meal at home with Nick and I; play with toys in the lounge; bathed by his father before bed. He did, however, still have two rather exhausted parents!

CHAPTER 19

Another summer

The summer of 1997 was now upon us and I tried my best to make the best of every day at home with my son. Yet I knew with each day that passed my inevitable return to work was coming closer, probably in September, which I would have to face along with all the pressures of life I had crumbled under in previous months. My appointments continued with the psychiatric nurse, whom I now saw just at the hospital; the consultant, who listened to my progress; my GP, who kept prescribing the antidepressants; and the health visitor, who noted at her visit in mid-May that she had seen Dominic at home in his highchair, eating and using a cup. He was mobilising well around furniture and there were plenty of age-appropriate toys and a play pen. He was vocalising, saying 'tick-tock' and 'No', with lots of smiling. I think she must have been happy with us.

In early May the local education office referred me to the County Medical Advisor who had been informed of my prolonged period of sickness and wanted to see if there was any way in which she could be of assistance. The letter expressed concern, rather than a threat, which was appreciated at the time. It was sensitively put together and stressed that the aim of the meetings were to help, if possible, a speedy return to health and work. The service was to act as a communication bridge between me, my doctor and school management, by offering advice and help, such as providing extra funding for me to work part time and have additional support. I consequently saw this doctor who reassured me that my return would be monitored and, in the meantime, to continue making a full recovery. I tried to resume a 'normal' lifestyle again and arranged a whole range of ways to spend my recuperation. Part of me still longed to be just in my dressing gown, staying in and being 'safe'. Yet the continual battle and pressure to be a working mother was forever on the horizon with a sense of urgency and thus I put unnecessary pressure upon myself to keep busy, to cope, to maintain a clean and tidy home, to look immaculate with an equally squeaky-clean baby. All this linked with the guilt I still felt at times and the worry of being 'seen' out and about whilst on sick leave. Yet all these outings I saw as my recovery and had to hope society would understand. Little did people know the continuing personal monitoring I undertook each trip. It seemed there were three of me at times – the big person in the middle who moved and spoke to the outside world but who was constantly being praised or criticised by mini-Elaines on each shoulder. One would be telling me how well I had just coped, like driving the car, only to be interrupted by the other doubting I could then cope in the theatre, for example. Yet I continued to push myself along.

As a couple, socially our diary filled a little with more cinema trips and a barn dance in the church hall with Sue and Jon. I felt relaxed and it was good fun plus I was pleased that I coped with all the people. We stayed one night at Roy and Beverley's in Leeds where we had a Midsummer's Night Christmas meal to make up for what we had missed! When Dominic woke at 3 a.m., Nick was still up drinking malt whisky with Roy. However, there were still a few invitations I declined with people I did not feel close to and could not handle their questioning looks and awkwardness. Nick and I had a night in a hotel at Betwys-coed over Whitsuntide weekend. We had a lovely meal and for once I abandoned all thoughts of calories. After we had eaten we went for a walk, as it was a balmy night. Romantically we walked hand in hand and tried to convince each other that our life together was not so bad after all. I then had to make a dash for the grotty local toilets – the rich food was too much for me – and there was no toilet paper! Our climb up Snowdon the next day was better and I felt the exhilaration of fresh air, adrenaline and pleasure at being a couple. We bought Dominic a cute baby fleece. My parents' encouragement for us to spend time together like this was a good thing. They enjoyed having Dominic, he loved being with them and we got a break we needed. We spent our second wedding anniversary at the Craxton Wood Hotel and had a delicious meal. I managed to wear my 'hen-night' outfit (a sexy, backless number) and felt quite good. The *maitre-d* spoilt us and it was a success. At least I was thinner than last year and did not have leaking breasts!

We had a birthday barbecue at our house with friends, neighbours and my parents, which was a successful night even though we were in the garage due to the rain! Everyone laughed when Beverley encouraged the children to reorganise Nick's precious collection of magnets on the big fridge in the garage. He is renowned for being house proud and particular. I tease him for his obsessive behaviour at times and say he has autistic tendencies!

Although I had begun to relax a little more, Nick seemed annoyed and irritated with Dominic when we went out. He seemed to resent that his peace had been shattered. These days I would tell him to 'chill'. Back then I was so glad of his continuing support that I did not have the confidence to criticise him. Yet it was usually my fault we were out. I insisted we should still go out and no one said 'No' to me either! One Sunday we had lunch out with my family. It was at a traditional, small and smart hotel where the older, affluent people of Manchester dine. Therefore with a restless one-year-old it was not easy to relax for fear of us potentially disturbing other diners. Nick was on edge and so was I. My mother watched my every expression. The food was good but it was very stressful. Another time we returned with Nick's family for Patrick's 18th birthday, gluttons for punishment. It was much quieter though and Dominic was much happier exploring a whole array of food on his highchair tray. He had also learnt to look up in the sky for aeroplanes, which could be heard regularly.

Some trips together as a family of three were a success, e.g. a day out to Ness Gardens on the Wirral; early evening bike rides in Delamere Forest; lunch at Diane and Jon's, my friends from college. A walk and snack at Arley Hall and gardens was good too. It was quiet with space for us to wander. We let Dominic crawl on some of the lawn and both tried to hide from him. Simple actions but good, healing ones. It is true that a smile can heal. He got a paddling pool for the back garden and on sunny days we all had fun watching him with it. He had a very cute habit of waving the hose pipe and telling us it went 'oooo'. It became clear that a son/father bond was developing. Dominic crawled around one morning at home looking for his 'Dad' but he was at work. Another night when Nick was late home due to a school trip he refused to sleep until he had seen him. Nick began to buy him small presents from visiting salesmen at school, for example he bought him a musical toothbrush which he loved. Dominic had become more mobile and liked to 'help' outside. His favourite trick was to crawl underneath the dripping hanging basket when Nick had watered it! He would also sit in his swing to watch Nick cut the grass. We both did lots of planting and gardening. It was a good summer, weather wise, that year. We had the new car and were both pleased with it. It was a plush model and had been well cared for. We got bike racks for the roof and were determined to have a few family rides – part of the fitness and 'let's try to be a happy family' campaign.

I managed to do some things we could not have if I was working, for example Dominic and I went to the Cheshire Show with my parents. I felt really like a skiver there. At the time my parents were going through their own crisis and their problems somehow made me feel stronger because they needed *me* this time. Dominic relished the attention we all gave him and we ended the day successfully with an Italian meal in Knutsford where the cries of a tired baby did not matter in a bustling, family restaurant. I continued to take my grandparents for hospital appointments which usually ended up taking all day by the time we had waited, been attended to, had lunch and shopped for their groceries.

Dominic and I continued many activities as 'mum and son' that summer. I even ran an NCT coffee morning – at our house! We got a gazebo and I coped with six mums plus babies and toddlers. We went on trips to Gulliver's World and to Chester Zoo with Mums and Tots. I felt proud of Dominic that day as he was pleasant and cute. For once it was a few other children who were demanding instead of mine. It was a shame that other people's struggles gave me strength!

Another sunny day just the two of us went to Walton Gardens, where we had a picnic, looked at animals, cuddled on a rug and devoured ice cream. It was a lovely day when I can honestly say I truly felt that I loved my baby unconditionally. I was relaxed and we just enjoyed each other's company. I had begun to feel proud when complimented by strangers on his looks and behaviour. He had taken his first steps over the summer and got his first real shoes. He first said 'Mummy' on 31 July and two days later he said 'Grandma' at a barbeque at my parents. There were the young, 'normal' families of their best friends there that evening and it was the first time in a few weeks that I had felt awkward and embarrassed about my illness, so I kept quiet.

Although I kept busy, not every trip was good and most were not easy. Dominic and I went to Jeannie's antenatal class reunion. It was a lovely sunny day and we all sat in the perfect back garden full of new outside toys. I remember being overloud and chatty to compensate for my strong feelings of inadequacy and failure again. Two of the other mothers were now back at work part time as a doctor and lawyer. Why could they cope and yet not me? Everyone else was wearing appropriate summer outfits, but I had leggings, jumper, waistcoat and boots on. I could not even dress properly. They were all very kind to me and part of me enjoyed it. Unfortunately the other part wanted to run away and cry and cry. I did when we got home. Dominic got sunburnt arms and cheeks. I could not even protect him from the sun. My own class reunion was a little easier at my own health centre, but why did everyone else's baby sleep? We continued to be disturbed several times a night again. We also went to a big gathering at the health centre for a sponsored lunch for breast-feeding awareness week. Again I felt lonely in a big room; I did not speak to all these smiling happy mothers and asked myself why had I been the one with all the problems. What had I done to deserve it? I look at some photographs now of Dominic at this age and can ache for the strong desire to feel him in his tactile, cuddly clothes; the smell; the gurgles. I feel so very sad that at the time I did not fully appreciate it because I was too preoccupied with coping with life, especially me and how I was feeling. In photos I look fine but underneath I was still analysing every mood, outing, and potential visit, all with the eternal ticking of the 'back to work' clock. It still scared me but I had to return.

The health visitor suggested we began another sleep chart for Dominic in early July to try to find any patterns or possible causes. We still only had the occasional good night and Nick and I rarely slept together. Dominic still had irregular day naps but I had learnt to rest more with him, even if I watched daytime television. I would talk out loud to convince myself that I did not have to tidy up, faff around in the study with post, do the ironing, etc., but to stop and relax. Nothing seemed to work though with his sleeping and during one waiting period with my grandparents in Chester hospital I found an article about an osteopath who claimed that many children suffer behavioural and sleep problems due to pressures and stress in their skull and spine, possibly caused by an awkward birth. By massaging their skulls she claimed to have helped many children. I was excited by such claims and even though the rest of the family were sceptical, I took him along. She listened to our history and eventually examined him and did indeed manipulate and massage his skull and said she had found areas of tension. That night he slept through! In the end I took him for a few appointments and felt they did some good. Nick thought we were just throwing money away. It made me realise why parents will go to any lengths to help 'cure' their children of physical or health problems. If someone appears to offer a lifeline you feel compelled to take it.

Dominic had carried on spending some time each week with Cathy with a view to him going full time from September. The days to myself enabled me to do all the house chores and look after myself. I still mainly slept during them. I called into school a few times for brief visits but always took Dominic as a distraction from me. I still felt very guilty about every aspect of the previous year. In early July I went to a careers exhibition for schools. I actually began to buzz with optimism for work again as I talked about redeveloping work experience links for my pupils again and the 'old' me shone through. I also saw a colleague from another school there, Larry, who always makes me feel good! Maybe everything would be alright. All of us concerned decided I should attend school officially for each Friday in July and a few days during the last week of term. This would enable me to think about my planning, get used to being at work again and help me cope better with the prospect of returning properly in September. Although I felt I really wanted to resume my post, part of me was still very concerned that I might not be ready. I was only just beginning to handle everyday life and the prospect of full-time work was a huge mountain still to climb. I certainly wanted to give it a try.

I continued to make steady progress and achievements over the summer of 1997. It was lovely to have Nick around every day and we prepared for our holiday. We had chosen a cottage in the far northwest of Scotland for a week and I had thoroughly enjoyed planning our journey there and back, when we would stop off at a number of bed and breakfast places en route. When we had booked them it was with the hope that of course Dominic would be sleeping well by then. In reality, the B & B nights were terrible! Being cocooned in a small room with a noisy toddler is not a good idea when walls are so thin and you are concerned that you will disturb other guests. We had begun to ignore Dominic if he woke at night at home and if he was content to amuse himself then so be it. Unfortunately when he spotted us in the B & B bedrooms, he thought we were there to play! Added pressures arose at mealtimes because they either did not have a highchair or, if they did, it had no reins, tray or was broken. A minor detail maybe but if Dominic could not sit safely to eat then it was a problem. It was annoying as I had booked the places which advertised themselves as 'child-friendly' with appropriate equipment, yet they only provided a token gesture.

Our cottage at Lochinver was beautiful and only a short distance from idyllic beaches, where we spent many hours relaxing and playing. I have many fond memories of Nick and Dominic walking hand in hand along the shoreline, finding simple pleasures in the waves breaking and stopping to study a piece of floating seaweed, for example. Watching them together made me optimistic that maybe one day we would be the close, happy family that I had always wanted. Prior to the trip I had researched the recommended places to visit and eat at in the area. In retrospect, when I look at all the many places we went to that week, it is hardly surprising we were both so very tired. Just as a couple it would have been hectic, but with a very energetic toddler it was madness! However, we had come a long way from my New Year in hospital and we were both grateful. Nick had always wanted to explore this part of Scotland and I guess I wanted to organise us seeing and doing as much as possible to prove to him that we could do such things as a family. Why did I exhaust us in the process though? On the whole we did enjoy the holiday and drank a bottle of champagne on our last night in the cottage.

We had planned to drive home again over three days, stopping at more B & Bs. The first night's stay was acceptable as we had a large room with three beds and a cot in it, and we knew that there were no neighbours to disturb. The second night we had just settled Dominic to sleep in our tiny room only to have him disturbed by the bathroom and toilet trips of some Japanese tourists! He then only went back to sleep when we did at midnight. At 3.45 a.m. he was awake again, making his hosepipe and vacuum cleaner noises, ready to play! At least we had begun to laugh at such events as anger would have been futile. We made a cup of tea and just after 4 a.m. we came to the mutual decision of 'let's go home – now!' Within half an hour we had packed up and after having disturbed the owners to tell them we were going (bet we were popular!), we set off south, behaving like giggling, truanting school children! We drove through a deserted Glencoe in the moonlight. Dominic was still being a hosepipe as we spotted a stag in the distance, with small lochs and islands draped in the mists. It was a beautiful, exciting journey where we felt like the only people in Scotland and it was almost a mystical end to our holiday. In spite of everything, we were still good friends and I had survived it all. By 11 o'clock we were home and began to unpack in our usual efficient, Hanzak style, and by the time we sank into our (separate) beds there was hardly a trace we had been away!

My confidence was boosted even higher the following week when I stayed one night with a college friend of mine, Carole, just outside

Birmingham, with Dominic. She had been one of the people with whom I had corresponded whilst I had been in hospital and it was great to actually meet her again and to thank her for her support at that time. We met up with Claire the next day and went to a Baby and Toddler show at the National Exhibition Centre. I was really pleased with myself as I had driven on unfamiliar and busy roads on my own with Dominic. I had been sociable, although I am not sure what my friend's husband thought of me as I recalled my previous few years! I managed the crowds at the exhibition with no panic attacks, even though the risk was high. Just before our return home we had a spaghetti tea at the Pizza Factory in Birmingham where Dominic was treated as a star with plenty of attention, clean and appropriate equipment, and even toys to play with – a real child-friendly place. I commented to Claire that my baby was now definitely a toddler as he made patterns with his spaghetti (strange that it made vacuum cleaner noises too!). I told her I was quite prepared for school and felt confident and ready to try it. We had built up his time at Cathy's where her two boys were good with him and he liked their company too.

I could now drive again, organise myself and others, cope in crowds, make conversation and was surely better now, wasn't I? On holiday I had bought a few games for my class and treated myself to some new school clothes. The child-minding situation was not a problem and I anticipated the return to a routine with optimism. The doubting Elaine who kept muttering 'Not yet, not yet – you're still not sleeping, you're still on medication' was ignored. I was going back to work and that, quite simply, was that.

CHAPTER 20

Back to school

On my first day back after the summer holidays, Dominic had to be woken up and taken to my parents in his pyjamas for his breakfast. It was one of the few times we had ever needed to wake him – typical! Once at school I felt very, very nervous. People I had known for years seemed almost uncomfortable to be with me and worried about what to say to me. I was very glad of Nick being around but we try to keep a distance from each other at work. How I wanted to hold his hand for reassurance like I had done on many occasions in recent months. At least there were no pupils and we had some training instead. We listened to a speaker in the hall but I could not concentrate for my mind whirring about the bodies around me. I went in the small staff room at coffee break but felt the beginnings of a panic attack so wandered the corridors in tears instead. Yet I stayed the rest of the day in spite of feeling sick, headachy and generally as though I was tied in knots. I could not wait to get home and busied myself making a meal for us and my parents when they brought Dominic home. We had a family playtime before bed.

The next day we had more training. I was much more relaxed and coped better but was very grumpy for part of the evening back at home. We had left Dominic at Cathy's where he had had a good day. Both he and I were awake from 4.30 a.m. for an hour and of course were deeply asleep when it was time to get up. Luckily the third day at school was for preparation. The occupational health team had arranged that I could job share initially. I was to have two and a half days in school when I would be shadowed by another teacher, who would take over in my absence. The young teacher concerned had not really taught in special schools before so in explaining activities and ideas I felt some of my old confidence return. I used to give presentations about this class, so why was it so hard to tell just one person? I felt reasonably in control and happy with the arrangements. Part of me felt pleased to be back in my old surroundings and I tidied up and put things back to how I used to have them before my absence. It felt good! Teaching these youngsters had given me so much more personal determination to succeed and be assertive in the past and I was optimistic for it again. From school I went to see my GP and recalled my feelings on returning to work. She praised me but said she would continue to closely monitor and help me.

Sensibly we had decided to relax over the weekend. The whole country was actually grieving at this time due to the tragic loss of Princess Diana and I spent Saturday watching her funeral. Some of the tears I shed that day were a good release for me in many ways and I felt it was quite ironic that she too had suffered from postnatal illness. Many people believed she had everything too and what did she have to be miserable about? I never understood then either, but I do now. Nick took Dominic to see his family the next day whilst I did some planning for school for the first time in months. It was quite nerve wracking. Later we went out with my family for a meal.

I took Dominic to our church coffee morning on the Monday, as I felt we were now really on the last lap of such visits. After lunch I dropped him at Cathy's and I went to school. I was very worried about seeing the pupils again but got on with teaching. To observers again I probably seemed fine, but in reality I felt sick, had a headache and my heart was pounding. Some of the pupils were lovely and their enthusiasm and affection did help to motivate me to carry on. My 'shadow' teacher, assistant and I discussed plans with the group for the forthcoming term and there was an air of optimism. At times I felt myself being overbearing and loud to compensate for my huge feeling of inadequacy. At the end of the day I sat in the staff room for a meeting. I still really did not feel comfortable in this room. I stayed initially but had a panic attack as it filled up, so left.

Next morning I did a hospital run with my grandparents and Dominic (silly me). Once again I told everyone I was fine to do it. 'Make the most of it,' I told my mother, 'whilst I am still available.' My grandparents though did not appreciate my sense of urgency to get back in time for work as they ambled around a supermarket after the appointment. Consequently I arrived at my class stressed due to being late. When I collected Dominic from Cathy's later he showered me with kisses which felt great. Next morning I decided to take it easier and as it was sunny I packed us a little picnic which we ate in the local park before we separated for the afternoon again. I did not mind this aspect, it was where I was going that bothered me. I got through the following afternoon and thought it was getting a little easier. It was all the staff and pupils I found hard, not the actual tasks or planning. I went to see the film *The Full Monty* with friends that night and chuckled to myself for hours!

Next day I was in school all day. It was our minibus outing and as part of our leisure activities and mathematics we went to play crazy golf. I was very nervous about the whole trip but enjoyed the success of one of my pupils which consequently lifted my mood. We went back to school for lunch but yet again I could not face going into the staff room so chatted with the head teacher at the dining table instead. Naturally she was concerned how I was getting along and I was reasonably honest with her in my 'exterior' optimistic way. When I got home after school I went to bed, had a sob and forty winks, which was my way of dealing with the tiredness I was feeling. Later I went to a keep fit class and the adrenaline rush helped me to improve. The most obvious change in me since returning to school was the marked deterioration in my sleeping habits again. I had returned to 'normal' towards the end of the holiday but now I was back constantly in the spare room every night, very restless and thrashing about. I was having nightmares of running and running down never-ending corridors, banging my head against walls, and thus waking up in a panic.

The following week I decided I needed to sort out my wardrobe regarding suitable work clothes and on Tuesday ended up going to Marks and Spencer to try some more. We had lunch there before I dropped Dominic off at Cathy's and went into school. I felt tired all afternoon and thought the session dragged and that the class were bored with me. This led to a huge drop in my mood. I wanted to see the head teacher but she was too busy, so I collected Dominic and returned to school. I tried to explain that I was feeling very ruffled and beginning to struggle. She listened sympathetically, pointed out my successes so far and said that she hoped my mood would lift again. At home I tried to relax during the evening, but could not. By bedtime I lay on the bed very upset, about nothing specific, just everything. I felt I could not cope. I was swimming against the tide, like a hamster in a wheel. I was swamped by all I had to do. I realised I had struggled before and overcome 'mountains', but this one felt so *very* steep with a sheer drop down the other side, back to hospital. I felt like I was hanging on by my fingernails. I eventually slept in the spare room, rocking myself. I had self-harmful thoughts again for the first time in months. I wanted to be in hospital where it was safe. After a fitful few hours' sleep I was awake from 4 a.m. to 5.30 a.m., mulling all these fears over again and again.

Next morning I left Dominic in his cot while I got ready, as I could not cope with him. We went to Sue's as I felt she understood a bit, but basically I felt very lonely in this. Everyone tried to say the right thing, e.g. 'Everyone feels stressed/tired', but they were not cutting themselves last December. Leaving Dominic was not a problem, but I was. I realised I needed help but also felt a failure. I was being stupid. I was making a big fuss over nothing. I attempted to do positive things to help myself. I arranged to see my psychiatric nurse; told my assistant and 'shadow' teacher that I needed more help; chatted to other staff. I did want to cope and wanted to stop this slide back down to self-abuse, exhaustion and the inability to relax. I wanted to 'blank out'. Indeed I felt myself doing just that whilst driving and just staring. I had put a big face on, put my best foot forward, but I was faltering.

Back at home I resorted to more 'self-help' techniques by identifying my strengths and weaknesses and making a plan:

Positive

- Been to school as arranged.
- Taken some sessions quite well in spite of inner anxieties.
- Organised college, run off letters, answered post.
- Stayed in Monday and Wednesday staff meetings.
- Worked at home most nights on something.
- Kept up Keep Fit.
- Trying to get help.
- Had spells of enjoyment and success.

Negative

- Feeling swamped by all that is expected of me within two and a half days – how on earth can I cope with five?
- Drowning under all pressures waiting for me, e.g. rewriting the school Personal, Health and Social Education curriculum.
- Other staff planned every session, etc. – I have done overall plan but that is it. Cannot face setting individual objectives for my pupils.
- Worry about what to wear.
- Am I being stupid?
- Want to run away and drive and drive.
- Beginning to feel I am shutting down from physical contact with nearest and dearest again – did not want usual hug from parents.
- My head is spinning, like being drunk. I want it to stop.
- Scared of going to sleep as I am so restless and have horrid dreams.
- So scared that I have dropped so low so suddenly. I realise it is not going to be up and up but did not expect a down to be so very low down. Finding 'comfort' in thinking how to hurt myself again, e.g. cutting, stabbing, overdose, nightdress wander. The urge is so very strong. Where have I gone? I thought these thoughts had disappeared but obviously they have not.
- Sleep!!

The best plan that night was to go to sleep. I had shared many of these thoughts with Nick and at last I went to sleep in our bed with the strict instruction that I was not to get up in the night to Dominic. After an hour of unsuccessfully getting him back to sleep at 3 a.m., I heard doors slam and the car start up. Nick spent the next hour driving round and round the area to try to get him off again, to no avail. I think it was fair to say that the father/son relationship was somewhat strained at this point.

I coped reasonably well the next day at work and felt more optimistic again as I faced another three-day weekend. I had another 3 a.m. session with Dominic. In retrospect, I wonder if he sensed the change in me? He was tired the next couple of days, culminating with a very unsuccessful

Tumble Tots (a gym club for toddlers) trip with Nick as he moaned the whole time. My parents sprung to the rescue and took him out for the rest of the day, leaving us time to relax. I did some school work! We all had a better night and had a pleasant day out with my parents on a walk around Tatton Park and tea in an Italian restaurant where Dominic had a great time exploring a plate of long spaghetti. The sunshine, fresh air and generally relaxed day left us all refreshed and ready to battle on.

I went to see my GP next morning and although I told her my thoughts from last week, I now said I was fine and just asked for more antidepressants. Since my return to work I had become very aware of when their effect was wearing off and I definitely did not want to stop them. I told her I was due to see the county occupational health doctor on Friday. My GP said she also wanted to see me then. Oh dear. I pushed all negative thoughts aside again and had lunch with Sue and denied all the feelings I had shared with her last week. I was going to be fine now, no problem. My mother was due the next day to have an operation on her leg, so she insisted that they should have Dominic that night for us as she would be having several days in bed after that. I reluctantly agreed because I was fine, wasn't I? I managed the next two half-days and a full day quite well in class, surviving on bravado and 'I am not going to fail again' vein. Meanwhile the usually well-behaved Dominic had bitten Cathy's hand when she had chastised him for something! Maybe he was sensing the tension surrounding us?

My appointment with the county doctor arrived and I took myself confidently to Chester. I sat in the waiting room, praising myself for the progress I had made so far. I was working again. Only a few months ago I had been a psychiatric patient having electric shock treatment. When called in I told her how well I was doing with the two and a half days. My separation from Dominic was fine and I was pleased he was happy at his childminder's. I chatted incessantly about my plans for my group and how I wanted them to progress. I was bubbly and on a high. Almost as an afterthought I told her how I had felt last week but that all that was over now. She put her pen down. She took a long sigh, looked me straight in the eye and slowly said, 'I'm very, very sorry. I can see you have tried your best and that you want to succeed to please everyone, including yourself, but I really have to forbid you from going back to school.'

I just stared back, feeling I had been slapped hard.

'You see,' she continued, 'in my role, if someone tells me, as you have just done, that they want to harm themselves as a result of being in their place of work, I have to deny them from returning until they are fully fit. In my opinion you are not yet fully fit. We could look at options for you retiring on grounds of ill health but your pension would be minimal and I feel that you will probably be fit again one day – just not yet.'

She told me she would write to my head teacher to inform her of her decision, along with the recommendation that I did not return until just before the Easter holidays, in five months' time. She felt this would give me a clear goal to aim for, which was realistic, but also would enable school staff to plan accordingly rather than lurch along on fortnightly sick notes. I numbly thanked her. She shook my hand warmly. I left. I walked in a daze through the crowded streets of Chester and at last found a phone box. I dialled the school number. Nick answered the phone.

'I'm a failure again,' I mumbled. 'I've been forbidden to work. I'm a threat to myself and to the Education Authority for the risk I pose.'

He obviously was disappointed. He so much wanted a 'routine' and normal life again. Once again it was being taken from us. When I got back to the car I held the steering wheel tightly and howled. Why us? Why me? Why does everyone else cope with life and I cannot? My heart was heavy and my stomach in knots as I drove back to Runcorn.

I hardly spoke to my GP, who did not seem surprised by the outcome of the meeting and tried to lift my spirits, to no avail. My mother began my road to recovery again, when we visited her in hospital later that evening, as she pointed out that it meant I had more time to myself and with Dominic. Five months seemed like a long period at this stage but in the grand plan of life it was a short time. She told me to think back five months and compare the state I was in now to then, which on the whole was a huge improvement. So maybe she was right and in another five months' time I probably would be much more ready than I was now.

Yet we did have a new routine, but it was just one that we had not planned. Nick was at work full time. Dominic went to Cathy's on Monday, Tuesday and Wednesday afternoons plus all day Thursday and Friday. I looked after him at other times and I was supposed to relax and recover the rest of the time. Dominic was happy with his routine. At Cathy's he would go to and from the local school for her boys; played with other toddlers and older children also minded by her after school and they went to Mums and Tots church groups three times a week. I was pleased he mixed with children of other ages and was not clingy with me. Yet another diary started, written by Cathy to describe his antics. She noticed several aspects of Dominic's character which are still evident a few years later – sociable, affectionate, a good dancer, left-handed, very vocal and chatty. He liked cheese sandwiches, grapes, yoghurt and pasta and was not a big drinker. He varied from a model child, being cute, intelligent and well behaved, to being demanding, whingy and grumpy, usually as he was tired and refused to sleep. Cathy could not figure out his aversion to sleep and declared he was the worst child she had known for it! At least it was not just us who thought that. We had to make a 'one-hour nap rule' in the hope he may sleep better at night, but it did not make much difference as he still disturbed us most nights.

I was mainly back to sleeping in the spare bedroom again so that I would not wake Nick with my nocturnal habits and so I could be on duty for Dominic, sometimes two and three times. Nick was on duty at weekends, me in the week. Often all he needed was his bottle of water handing to him and he would go straight off again. Without the bottle he could be awake for hours, so it was the easiest option. A couple of times the bottle leaked all over the cot, needing the bedding to be fully changed. Occasionally he would find it himself and after a couple of sucks he would settle, so we thought it was worth persevering with. He still refused a dummy. His days were so busy yet they still did not wear him out. I was the one who continued to be exhausted and in my 'free' time I often slept. If I had been really disturbed on a Sunday, Monday or Tuesday night, Nick would take Dominic to my father for the morning so I could catch up on a few hours' sleep. On Thursday and Friday mornings I would get Dominic ready for Cathy's and when he and Nick left I would continue to take the papers and post back up to bed and not emerge until almost lunchtime. At last I was learning to sleep again, even it was at the wrong times. I even had afternoon naps on the settee, a habit I had never had before. I became a daytime television viewer and especially liked the morning 'magazine' programmes. Curled up in my dressing gown I felt that the presenters were my friends each day, such as 'Richard and Judy', and looked forward to the programmes. Often I would sympathise with viewers who called for help with their problems, which gave me comfort that there was not only 'me' going through a difficult time. I had visions of many others in their dressing gowns! 'Success' features of people who had come through adversities were inspiring and I longed to be on that side of my current situation.

All my appointments with the health professionals continued and my diary most weeks involved one or two of them. A week did not pass without at least one home visit or me sitting in a waiting room somewhere. I particularly liked my meetings with my CPN and liked to talk freely about how I was progressing or otherwise. I felt I could tell him anything. I had been told in hospital that initially I was having all bad days with the occasional good one. They suggested that little by little the good days would improve and the bad times decrease. Generally I was improving but still had bad days when my zest for life was non-existent and I was tearful and lethargic. I learnt to accept these and just ride it out by sleeping and lazing around. Often the next day I would wake full of the joys of spring and whizz around doing everything and anything. Without any pressure on me I was able to adapt my activities to my status and learnt to say 'no' if I did not feel up to doing something. Pushing myself made me worse later on so it was not worth it.

At weekends we tried to be 'a family' and did get out and about. One favourite outing was a 'show house fix'. When we had been house hunting we looked at some and subsequently for ideas in our own home. We enjoyed it and carried on looking. Dominic thought it was good fun crawling up the stairs and especially liked to try to turn on taps. He began to think it was perfectly normal to look around houses, to explore them top to bottom and criticise them! We had pleasant days out with friends on the Welshpool railway for a Postman Pat day and a pub lunch and train ride at Rudyard Lake. We went to the Blackpool Illuminations where Dominic liked walking along the tableaux and saw Postman Pat and Thomas. His favourite was a huge peeping worm. We had chips in the street (why do they taste so good outside?) and drove through the rest with a running commentary from Dominic. A success! A happy family at last?

We spent half-term at another time-share apartment my parents had booked and let us use. We had a two-bedroom apartment in a tiny village called Little Haven, on the Pembrokeshire coast, and had some happy times. In the week or two prior to going away I had set myself a project making a guide book on the area, compiled from tourist information leaflets and recommended guides. I knew the area well by the time we went and had a file with all the copied references in it. I found such tasks very therapeutic. Dominic was hard work as he wanted to be on the go the whole time, even when he was obviously tired and needed a rest. Sometimes I felt like 'piggy in the middle' as I tried hard to plan for places which I thought Dominic would like, but then if he was grumpy Nick would get impatient and irritated too. At such times I tried to keep the peace but equally felt cross with both of them and myself. We did have happy times though, mainly through observing Dominic's development. We were getting better at choosing child-friendly places and activities but still kept up too busy a pace considering the irregular sleep we all had.

Although we went out as a family, socially we had a minimalist approach. I did not want to go to a big party for a colleague who was 50 – still guilty that I should not socialise if I was off sick, but also because of all the 'crowds'. I went to some children's birthday parties with Dominic but I dreaded them still as it meant I had to make small talk with people. I continued to feel uncomfortable with people, finding 'simple' tasks a challenge. Each week I hated going in to collect Dominic from the Thursday Mums and Tots group as I felt (irrationally) everyone looked upon me as 'the loopy Mum who could not cope'. On the other hand I made progress by organising and running a book party one evening at home; a meal out with the Hanzaks for my mother-in-law's birthday and also had an evening with some former neighbours from my first marital home. The lady had always had a phobia about people being sick if she went out and had become more reclusive in recent years. Apparently I had become an inspiration to her and she had begun successfully to overcome it. She told me that watching me emerge from my illness had motivated her into doing something about hers! I was naturally pleased as I did not recognise any positive effects from my illness for anyone at this point.

I had learnt to overcome difficulties on a more regular basis, like panic attacks, and to try to find ways round them. For example, a year earlier Nick and I went to the theatre where I was terrified. I wanted to crawl behind the wallpaper and found the whole evening distressing. I now faced the challenge of seeing *Les Miserables* with my parents and Nick. We got there about 20 minutes early to avoid me panicking about being late and fighting through a crowded foyer. We found our seats and I suddenly thought, 'O-oh, I'm in a theatre again, first time since last Christmas.' At first I felt fine and felt my mood rise and rise to an unnatural level of exhilaration because I was not scared! Then people came and sat in front of us, behind us, around us, and I felt that panic, the tightening in my stomach feeling. Within minutes I was on the roller coaster ride of emotion but I weathered the storm by telling myself over and over again that I would be fine – and I was! We arrived back home to find Dominic in a dirty nappy watching *Newsnight* with my brother whom we had left babysitting!

I was still taking my antidepressants regularly but they did appear to cause a couple of frightening experiences for me, involving alcohol and a filling. Nick and I spent a very happy evening at Sue and Jon's, during which I discovered I needed an eye test. Recently I had noticed I struggled to read road signs at night and was convinced that the projectionist at the cinema had not focused the film properly. Eyesight cropped up in our conversation and I tried Jon's specs on – wow! What a difference. Within a few weeks I had my own for night driving and theatre/cinema trips. Jon commented to Sue later that evening that it was good to see a little sparkle back in my eyes again. This was the comment which later inspired this book's title! I drank several glasses of wine that night as it was the first time I had felt so inclined for a long time. When we got home I told Nick to go to bed as I was too restless. I just dropped on the spare bed, fully clothed, and said I would clean my teeth and undress a little later. Nick settled, and then I went into 'wild' mode and had a terrifying urge to hurt myself. I stumbled downstairs and grabbed a bottle of paracetamol. Part of my mind was telling me to stop being so stupid but the rest of me felt totally out of control. I suddenly needed to get fresh air and walked quietly out of the house, my head spinning. No shoes on again. I walked the dark and damp streets, not able to focus or walk straight. I was really scared. An hour previously I had been the life and soul at Sue's, now I was a crazed woman. I sat on some steps to try to think logically and for this madness in my head to stop. Next minute I opened the bottle of tablets and put a handful in my mouth. They tasted dry and disgusting so I spat them out into someone's front garden. I wandered further and repeated the pill taking and spitting out. I have no idea how long I was out but eventually I did find my way back home, had a huge drink of water, undressed and fell into bed. Next day I had a wicked hangover and felt very foolish and ashamed about my early hours' walk. Nick asked why my socks were wet by the washing machine! My GP explained that I should not have been drinking due to the antidepressants and that my five glasses of wine that night were the equivalent to about three bottles for someone not on that medication. No wonder my head felt 'pickled' that night. Yet nowhere on the leaflet with my pills did it stress the effects of mixing alcohol with them. I have since lost the desire to drink more than a few glasses at any time as I never want to feel like that again. It made me wonder if that is how drug users feel at times and, if so, I appreciate why they may do stupid and dangerous things under the influence.

Secondly, I had a bad reaction to a filling at the dentist. I am normally fine after one and it does not really bother me at all. However, as the local anaesthetic started wearing off, I just felt quite groggy and poorly. So I went to bed early, falling immediately into a rare, deep sleep until I woke up at 1 o'clock. The first thought in my mind was 'go in the nursery and smother Dominic!' Shocked and scared, I argued with myself that I definitely did not want to do that, then in the next instance the urge to stab myself arose. Suddenly I had this barrage of self-injurious thoughts and thoughts of attacking Dominic. I was very, very frightened and confused. Why was my mind doing this? Luckily I managed to stop myself from doing any of the actions I had thought of, and I ran to Nick, and pleaded, 'Quick, quick, give me a big hug! Give me a big hug, its horrible! Hold me tight and don't let me go.'

I explained and at last went back to sleep. I phoned both the dentist and the GP the following day and they thought maybe it could be a reaction with my antidepressants. I had felt my head was full of chemicals that were fighting each other. It frightened me though to feel that I was still on a slender line between being the logical, organised, busy, sensible person I wanted to be and being 'loopy' again.

I continued to fill my days with activities which made me feel good, such as keeping fit at the local class and at the village club. Sitting in the steam room after a good exercise session was very therapeutic. I helped with an NCT nearly-new sale, sorting and selling items. I continued to take my grandparents for appointments and care for them in general. On one shopping trip Dominic sucked the car keys and broke the car alarm, but I handled the dilemma well! I had another trip to the Merryhill centre and hotel with Dominic, my parents and Claire. We had fun in the pool; Dominic loved exploring the hotel foyer and Christmas tree and pretended to phone his father on the lobby phone. We all queued to see Father Christmas and had a family photograph with him. In spite of Dominic being awake from 2 a.m. to 4 a.m. with Claire and I, we were all much more relaxed than previous trips and enjoyed it.

Our weekend break had also given Nick some much needed time alone. I had time to myself when he was at school and Dominic at Cathy's but we made a conscious effort for Nick to 'escape', e.g. he went to a computer fair at Chester and stayed overnight at his friend's in Yorkshire. He and

Dominic still had a topsy-turvy relationship with peaks and troughs with little middle ground. Peaks were such as Dominic asking his father for a kiss and waving when he left for work. Troughs were at Tumble Tots where Dominic was still watching people instead of doing things, which Nick found frustrating; he had a short bath one night as he threw a whole jug of water over Nick. I was very aware how tiring and trying our lifestyle was for Nick and I felt guilty about it. To appease the situation I agreed at last that we should have a computer of our own, which he had been attempting to persuade me for a long time. We had often borrowed them from school but information technology was advancing fast and he felt we should be in the race. I was pleased to see him with his new 'toy', even though it was an expense we could not afford at the time.

I did not fully appreciate at the time how tremendously supportive Nick was to me and what a huge strain I must have been. His previous lifestyle as a bachelor, living alone for 12 years, had been changed out of all recognition. Our married life had presented challenges far beyond those we had anticipated but he approached them all with patience and resilience. All our pressures and problems did have a positive effect too, in that he had become much more tolerant and relaxed about everyday matters and very blasé about feminine wiles. It seemed my gender could surprise him no longer! One Sunday morning I was having a lie-in when the door bell was rung. Nick opened the door to be greeted by one of my friends sobbing hysterically and asking if I was in. It was raining. She had arrived by car, wearing only her night clothes and slippers! Nick suggested she would find me in upstairs. Cold and wet, I said she had better get in bed with me where I listened to her outpourings over her problems and we eventually succeeded in putting the world to rights. A little later Nick popped his head around the door to merely ask 'Tea or coffee?' At a later date she recalled that when Nick had originally opened the door to her that day, his reaction had been totally unruffled as he was obviously used to slightly crazy females!

One of our other problems was that financially we had lost around £6000 from my extended sickness leave which we have never recovered from, although it could have been much worse. Our generosity to each other had not helped, e.g. getting the computer, but at such times we needed treats too as compensation for the other stresses. On the Teachers Occupational Sick Pay scheme I was entitled to 100 days on full pay then 100 days on half pay. Whilst on half pay I could claim incapacity benefit, statutory sick pay and some help with child-minding fees. The application form was a nightmare. By going back for a few weeks in September it had put me back on to full pay again but we faced the new year on half pay. This added to my worries so I approached the Teachers Benevolent Fund (TBF), part of my teaching union. A very sympathetic local TBF secretary came to see me in November and said he would represent me at a local panel, but with no luck. They did offer a loan support scheme but I was also turned down for this. What happens to all the donations? Even a token gesture from my profession would have made a small difference.

I had finished all our Christmas shopping by the end of November; made Christmas cakes and cleaned the house enthusiastically. Dominic 'helped' me around the house with jobs and we played games as I worked. We put up the Christmas decorations with more pleasure than last year but had to discourage Dominic from taking them down again! I definitely now was enjoying time with him and would smile as he spent ages on simple activities such as amusing himself with an empty paste jar and lid. There was a mutual admiration developing now, judging by the photos, e.g. giggling and climbing into the pram folded in the hall with a sparkle in his eyes for me. I began to comment more often now on 'happy days' in the diary. We put his big pram away in the loft just before Christmas. I felt this was the end of an era. I did not want to sell any of his things just in case we ever had a second child. This was still a definite 'No' from Nick and also me at this stage, but I still had hope in spite of everything.

I was still bitter and disappointed about my experiences and little things still upset me. One night Dominic explored a frame and subsequently ripped up the photo from it of him and me when he was a newborn. I was heartbroken and decided that it summed up our whole sorry state. It was his way of showing me that he knew what a terrible mother I was and that I did not deserve him, let alone another child. I read a glowing article in a magazine one day about the joys of motherhood and sent the following letter, which shows the self-pity and anger I was feeling at the time.

24 November 1997

Dear Madam

'Aching to feel that maternal bond'

After reading 'A Secret Sensuality' and letter of the month (December SHE), I would ask you to spare a thought for those of use who do not instinctively feel a maternal bond with their child. All I ever wanted was to be a mother and after one unsuccessful marriage I was ecstatic to find myself pregnant a few months after my second marriage. The pregnancy was fine until seven months when I suffered a great deal of pain and many hospital stays due to kidney problems. The birth was horrific – the baby immediately taken from me as I was rushed off to theatre. The baby had suspected meningitis at 4 months old and never slept a full night until about a month ago – he is now 19 months old. I had been due back to my professional job as a teacher of disabled children the same week he was so ill but have not made it back since. Finally, last Christmas I had a total breakdown and spent weeks in a psychiatric hospital. Since then I have overcome suicidal feelings, panic attacks, severe mood swings and severe depression and am just beginning to live again. My son is at long last starting to become a real part of our lives but it has been so very, very hard. I do not feel guilty that this strong maternal bond has so far evaded me – just envious of those who do have it. No matter how very wanted a child is, it does not seem to me to guarantee the blissful, idyllic parenthood that I had always dreamed of.

This morning our son shouted 'mo-mmy' to me from his cot for the first time – my heart skipped a beat so maybe it's starting! We are determined this will be a very special Christmas.'

At the beginning of December I had to attend a meeting at our Local Education Office with my head teacher and authority officer to check on my intention to return to work. I felt that they had lost faith in me and although I did my best to say that I still wanted to work and that by March I would be ready, they seemed sceptical. The meeting did not upset me as I had learnt to live for the moment and school seemed miles away. Next morning I wrote all our Christmas cards. I won a local supermarket Christmas competition for food and a tree. Dominic and I had to collect the prizes and pose for the local newspaper. I felt very guilty when I saw the picture. What was I playing at? I looked brimming with health, confidence and happiness cuddling my little boy. The staff at work would really be convinced seeing this that I was indeed 'playing the system' and malingering. The side-effect of this was to dwell on my weaknesses for a few days to convince myself I was still not fit to work! I could not win. The dilemma of needing to be busy in order to learn how to cope clashed with guilt again on a trip to see Father Christmas. On one of my good days I decided to make the most of my time off and organised for a group of my friends with our toddlers to have a day out visiting a grotto and having lunch together. I was really excited about the trip until the party behind us in both the grotto and lunch venue were a class from my school! I wanted to crawl under the table. What a fraud! Another event I looked forward to was the NCT Christmas night out for a meal and dance at a local, small hotel. I did not feel I should go to the school event so this was my only chance for a dance and posh frock this year. All my exercise had paid off and I wore my backless, 'hen-night' dress and felt great. However, the night proved a total disappointment as all the entire group wanted to talk about was breast-feeding, toilet training and postnatal depression! When the disco started they complained it was too loud and moved into the lounge, so I did not even get a dance. These days I would have stayed by the music, but this is another indication that I was still not fully recovered.

Dominic woke when I got in and then I spent ages getting him to sleep again. At least it had been a good sign that I wanted to dress up, make small talk and dance, even if it did not go to plan!

In mid-December I was interviewed by a Masters student who was researching the possible causes of postnatal depression. I had answered a request for information from the support association and she had chosen me as one of her subjects. I recalled so many events to her that her tape ran out! I realised then that I quite liked talking about my illness. It seemed to help me begin to realise the trail of events which led to it and to recognise the progress I had made as our first proper Christmas as a family approached.

CHAPTER 21

Springtime

Christmas 1997 was very good, especially in contrast to the previous one I had spent in hospital. Dominic opened his presents in our bedroom and had to be coaxed into undoing them all. He wanted to play with each one fully before moving on to the next one. He liked the paper but also the presents, his favourites being cars, trains and 'Teletubby' items. Then Nick took him to my parents whilst we made the lunch for our families. One year on from my total breakdown I succeeded in planning, shopping, cooking and serving Christmas lunch and supper for ten people and loved every minute of it! We had even made a jazzy menu using our new computer. Even the socialising and chatting were no longer a strain and we all delighted in Dominic's continuing joy at opening yet more presents. His Auntie Claire won top prize for managing to have acquired the most hunted toy for that year – a cuddly 'Teletubby', from a television series. The day culminated in all of us watching a 'Teletubby' video! I had always enjoyed being a hostess prior to my illness and it now appeared that I could once again manage this aspect of life, with my closest family at least. I am sure they must have been relieved to see me handle the day well too. Boxing Day was happily spent with our neighbours and then visiting our respective families for more meals. We all look much more bright-eyed in the photographs this year. My comment in Dominic's diary was that it had been 'a nice Christmas'.

My mother and I had begun a new hobby of entering competitions wherever we saw them and were having some success. The day after Boxing Day we used our prize of a family ticket for Blackpool Tower. Nick stayed at home as Thomas the cat was poorly! Dominic, my parents and I had a great day and yet again my confidence was boosted by coping in crowds and busy places. The highlight was a 'Dawn of Time' ride which instigated Dominic's interest to this day in dinosaurs. New Year was also a colossal improvement upon the previous one. I decided I wanted to entertain again so Jon, Sue and the children came and we spent a very pleasant evening together. The children looked so cute snuggled up together in their nightclothes, appealing to my increasing maternal feelings for my son and god-daughter. After our meal the four adults posed for photographs using the remote setting. The smiles and warm hugs are almost impossible to relate to the previous year when I had been in hospital. There really is life after mental illness!

The rest of the holiday was spent at the sales, muddy walks in the local forest and seeing the family. All too soon Nick had to go back to work and the high I had been on all over Christmas lowered again. Likewise, just as all of our sleep patterns had begun to improve, Dominic was poorly again the first week of term with a rash, temperature and generally being niggly and restless. Yet again I was back to being disturbed several times a night and began to crumble. He was not well enough to go to Cathy's but luckily my father was around to give me a break. I think it concerned us all that there was still a fine line between me managing or not. We had a particularly bad Friday night/Saturday morning when he woke at 4.30 a.m. and could not settle again. By 6.30 a.m. he was being driven around the town in the car by his father and I was ironing! At least the next night was much better and we decided to wrap up warmly and headed to Llandudno for a few hours. The sea air and winds were exhilarating and watching Dominic's attempts to copy his father throwing stones into the sea was a tonic. The cuddly photographs of us that day again mask the utter strain of the previous morning.

We then managed to resume our pre-Christmas routines of Mums and Tots groups, shopping and socialising, still peppered with disturbed nights when Dominic would play the 'I'll wait until Mum and Dad have just gone back to sleep before I cry again' game. Most of the time we both coped reasonably well, but at other times we would feel cross, tired and upset as a result. Why, oh why did he not sleep like everyone else's child did? What did we do wrong? We attempted a 'let's get tough' regime, but this failed too. He managed to keep us sane by balancing a night from hell with him and then being a model child for us or Cathy if we went out. How could it be the same child? At his 20-month check with the health visitor our only concern was the continuing sleep problem. She noted that he 'walked well, climbs stairs, squats; built a three-brick tower; turned pages; scribbled; obeyed simple commands; said lots of clear words; identified several parts of the body'. She did, however, refer us back to the sleep clinic.

Two days later he had another excuse for being so restless and being awake almost every hour in the night – an ear infection! I wonder why Nick did not give him a kiss as he left for work that day? This episode was appeased by a couple of full, undisturbed nights. I could see Nick was beginning to look very tired again so decided to try to perk us all up by preparing a special candlelit tea. I smartened myself up too and tried to be chatty but he was just too tired to appreciate it. Dominic spent most of the weekend with his grandparents to give us some time together. They were very good at offering help when they could. Our batteries were recharged a little as we faced the next week. Dominic then had three days of being violently sick and ended up totally exhausted and lethargic. By the third evening he was admitted back into hospital with me on a folding bed at his side. Many of the staff remembered us!

He continued to be unable to keep fluids down and had to be put on a drip for 24 hours. That seemed to work but he was sick again all over me, the chair and floor a little later on. Luckily all I had to do was shout and a nurse came running and sorted us all out. A few hours passed and Dominic did begin to perk up so when the doctor came on his round he suggested he could go home. I burst into tears. The exhaustion again had made me feel very incompetent with all my mothering skills. I explained that I realised that my son was out of danger from dehydration, but pleaded that if they could spare our room for one more night then I probably would feel more confident to cope at home. I dreaded the thought of him being ill again all over me and not coping with the situation. I felt pathetic pouring out our saga since his previous hospital stay but tried to say I needed a little more help to get me through this bad patch. Luckily they listened to me and 24 hours later the same doctor found us both tucking into apple pie and custard with big grins on our faces! I had no hesitation for him to be discharged then and phoned for someone to collect us. It had to be my mother as Nick was now poorly in bed and remained there for a few days. Full marks to the paediatric team again!

Dominic improved and Nick went back to work. Later that week I took my grandparents for a hospital appointment. We waited ages for them to be seen which was not easy with a lively toddler. Then I took them for their groceries and suggested that they hurried if we were to have lunch out as planned because Dominic was due at Cathy's. Their version of 'hurry' differed from mine and so, extremely stressed, I got our meals in Marks and Spencer's café and dropped the tray with them on! I wanted to scream and yell at all the people who stared at me. At least the staff were helpful and soon sorted out the situation. Why on earth I did not just ring Cathy and not bother taking him I do not know – wisdom after the event!

The irregular night routines continued, some good nights, others were dreadful. In his diary for Cathy, one morning I wrote, 'Screams at 3.30 a.m. – left him. Screams at 6.45 a.m. – left him until he was quiet. We *will* win.' He once again made up for this by being very cute, well behaved and charming that evening when I took him briefly to a 21st birthday party of one of my former pupils. One of the other mothers from my support group was working behind the bar at the venue. It was good to see her 'surviving' again and she was amazed to hear that I had ended up in hospital the previous year.

Then we had the pleasure of my brother Kevin, Annie and Brendan visiting the UK again, staying at my parents. Kevin was going to be in Portsmouth for most of the time as he was still working on his PhD. This time I did not feel they were a threat in any way. Dominic and Brendan immediately got on well and it was good to watch them play together. My parents, Kevin, Annie, Brendan and us three all went to a time-share house at Kenmore in Scotland for half-term week. It was large and luxurious for us all and we had many successful family trips out to places of interest. My fundamental desire to 'make home' and subsequently 'keep house' was put to the test but I rose to the occasion and liked to cook and tidy after us all! I probably drove the rest of the family mad but it was ideal therapy for me. My parents loved spending time with their grandsons and it was good to see their relationship develop. Dominic began to be helpful, such as bringing his shoes to put on when asked, and even commented on happenings around him, e.g. 'Daddy's back!' His interest in new surroundings was fascinating to watch and the toddler stage of 'into everything' to learn about his environment also began to endear him more to both Nick and I.

Back at home he was developing an interest in all of his fathers' jobs outside and wanted to 'help' clean the cars. There were no problems until Nick let him hold the hosepipe which he promptly sprayed over the freshly dried and polished cars! Several times I had to intervene and try to balance Dominic's desire to copy his father with Nick's strictly routine-based tasks. An inquisitive toddler is not easy when you have had over 20 years of being your own boss in such tasks, but I had to try to convince him that time and patience was the key to the ultimate enjoyment of a team approach.

Over the next few weeks I became very aware that my time 'off' work was drawing to a close. In general I did feel far more confident about every area of my life and much stronger to cope mentally and physically with any knocks. I entered a 'make the most of it' period, arranging most days to meet up with my old and newer friends who had children, plus Brendan and Annie, and we all got out and about to a variety of places. I guess that Dominic's developing mobility, level of conversation and independent streak helped too. I did not feel I was leaving a helpless baby, but a boisterous toddler who definitely benefited from a wide range of company and venues. He had also begun to use a potty, very occasionally. I went into school to arrange with the head teacher about my return and it was decided that in the three weeks prior to the Easter holiday I would attend for three, four then five days, respectively. It was sensitively pointed out to me that this, understandably, was my last chance – fail this time and I was out.

A few days later I woke up feeling dreadful. I ached. I had a temperature. I was exhausted. After three days of just lying in bed incapacitated, my GP came to see me. She could not help but laugh at me! She diagnosed real influenza and said I would be fine within another week – just in time to go back to work! Her humour in my direction was that she simply could not believe my bad luck yet again with my health. After all my struggles in the last two years, here I was bedridden by an everyday but nonetheless debilitating virus just as I should have been enjoying my last days of freedom! I was so very worried that I would not be well enough physically by my deadline as I had been warned of the consequences.

Luckily I did perk up in time and a couple of days before I went back I arranged for a group of my closest friends, plus my mother, to go out for my 'going back to work' night out. We had a meal in a rather crowded and noisy restaurant. I felt so good to cope with that again and so grateful to those sitting with me for all the support they had given to get me back to this point with confidence.

My last weekend before I started back at school was quiet as my parents took Dominic and Brendan to the Holiday Inn at Maidenhead prior to Kevin and his family returning to Zimbabwe. They took the boys to 'Legoland', a place Dominic dreams about going to ever since! Meanwhile I began my first day back at work, minus my son to make it a little easier. I was very nervous and kept wanting to see Nick all day for an encouraging wink or smile. My new class was a very different environment to the situation I had left two years ago. Instead of the active group of 16–19 year-olds to whom I had been teaching independence skills, my new pupils were aged between seven and 16 with profound and multiple learning difficulties. Their physical needs were far beyond my previous experience and their level of understanding was also at a different level.

I had nine pupils with a team of three classroom assistants and several other supporting staff, such as midday assistants and medical professionals. There was nowhere to hide or be shy! Initially I wanted to tell my immediate staff why I had been off for so long as I felt they may not have gleaned the truth from rumours or lack of information. I wanted to ensure that they felt at ease with me and did not worry about upsetting me. For the first term I also taught two other classes over one day to give their teachers non-contact time to do administration work. Consequently in my first weeks back I was involved in three areas of school. Initially it seemed a huge challenge. I was mentally and physically exhausted but knew I had to survive. The staff were all very supportive and as the days went by my small successes began to grow, as did my ability to teach again.

In my first week I had two days off. The first I spent sensibly with Sue and her children, having fun at an indoor play area. We took our children too for a haircut. Dominic had his hair cut all over for the first time and sat quite well for the hairdresser. On the second day I had a morning at home and then a shopping trip with my grandparents. Dominic still was not sleeping well but this evening he actually bid me goodnight and there was not a peep all night. This gave me optimism! My assertiveness had also begun to return as in a shop a few days later an assistant unfairly told him off and I defended him strongly.

After a reasonable first week back we had another busy weekend. I had to take myself shopping to buy new clothes for school and actually got a few things which fitted me. The continuing exercises had paid off. We then had a fondue night for my parents, Claire and her boyfriend. I had also begun to risk the occasional glass of wine but after previous events did not touch much as I was still taking the antidepressants. Next day was Mothering Sunday. I was really pleased with the card and present Cathy had helped Dominic to make. After going to church I made all the family lunch at our house to celebrate Claire's birthday. My parents took Dominic to Chester Zoo so I could relax but I did some school work! I still seemed to have so much to prove by doing all this socialising and could never relax properly.

Not surprisingly the next day I went to bed straight from school! I remember too getting very upset as I took some of my pupils into the hydrotherapy pool. Seeing their fragile little limbs and how hard it was for them to bend stiff joints shocked and disturbed me. I was wracked with guilt that how could I worry about Dominic's lack of sleep, toilet-training saga and other 'problems' when the parents of these special children still faced such issues years later with probably no end in sight. Why could I not cope when these parents had continual dilemmas and crises to face? A huge wave of exhaustion, worry, stress and guilt was relieved by a long, deep cry and a big sleep that night. The next morning I felt refreshed to face the world again and vowed to try to keep my concerns in perspective. As a couple, Nick and I still had a lot going for us and we just had to keep on facing the hurdles together.

At the end of my second part-time week I had to report back to my GP and tried to convince her that I was managing reasonably well. The worse strain was that I took Dominic with me and he was mischievous, wanting to explore all the delights of her surgery. I felt that she would be thinking the classic comment that 'teachers' children are the worse'! In retrospect he was only being a typical toddler who was interested in a new environment. Still in busy, busy mode we spent that weekend with a trip to Gulliver's World theme park and visiting our families. On Sunday we attempted to clean, cook, iron, garden, clean cars and then went for a bike ride! All before my first full week back! Why did we have this manic obsession to be so busy? One reason was possibly to keep Dominic amused. He was so interested in everything around him and would be a danger to himself if left. It was therefore easier to keep on the move and provide him with plenty of stimulation.

My confidence in rearing Dominic was growing though, as evidenced by my advice to Cathy concerning his eating habits as she was struggling to expand his range of foodstuffs. I suggested various ideas but basically had a 'don't worry' approach as he may only pick at food for a few days then suddenly want to eat everything in sight. He did not pick between meals and we balanced what he did have. I ended my advice with 'If I'm wrong, please tell me!' She had two children of her own and minded many others. She said she worried more because he was not hers! Either way it was still good to be able to use Dominic's diary from her to chat about such things. Our nights were not as disturbed but he did tend to wake early, from

6 a.m. Often Nick would let me have an extra hour in bed, as I needed it, so he would feed and amuse him downstairs.

As we broke up for Easter I successfully managed a full working week involving three different classes. Although I had found it tiring I had managed most of the tasks quite well and felt confident enough to do some proper planning for my groups in the next term. The deputy head whose class I had taken over was still to share it with me until the summer so she still took most of the responsibility for everything. I just began to input my ideas where I could.

The Easter holidays began by my parents taking Dominic away for a few nights, again to give us time to relax or work. I had my hair unsuccessfully permed and had to go back a week later. It still did not 'take' as I wanted it too and I ended up with a semi-wild mess! It was most likely because I was still taking anti-depressants, which can affect the chemicals used by the hairdresser. My parents took Dominic to see *Snow White* at the Liverpool Empire with tickets they had won from the local newspaper. Sue said that she was getting worried that her godson never went anywhere unless it had been a prize! I went over to see one of my college friends who had just had a new baby. Not only did I cope with the sight of mother and baby but Dominic was so well behaved that it made the whole trip a pleasure instead of a stressful one.

My account of him in Cathy's diary after the holiday was that he had been lovely. He had slept well, eaten well and been well! He was now very polite to us and used some three-word phrases. It was a great relief to me that he had such an active and interesting time with her, which made my return to school easier. As a working mother, knowing that your child is well cared for and happy without you is invaluable. This was one worry I did not have as the summer term commenced.

CHAPTER 22

Back to reality

At last we had a proper routine with both Nick and I at work Monday to Friday and Dominic going to Cathy's. My parents helped us out on Monday and Wednesday afternoons when we had staff meetings. They collected him from Cathy's and took him home for a meal with them. Not only did this mean that we did not have to panic about being late but it also gave us two early evenings alone together. As a family we would also all go for a meal sometimes in the week for which we were grateful. Dominic settled well back at Cathy's and I actually succeeded with being back at work full time! I felt that everyone was watching me for any signs of weakness, not in a vindictive manner, but out of concern. For just over two years now I had been a worry for my nearest and dearest but also in my profession and with my colleagues. I continued to portray an exterior of confidence (I think!) but at least underneath I was actually beginning to feel it too. My desire to want my working environment well organised and tidy was initially too strong as I used it unknowingly and unintentionally as an excuse not to actually work with the children. It was a way of feeling that I was in control of something but I also acknowledge that I simply like being tidy regardless of any analysing! The staggered return had worked well and as the weeks passed in school my confidence, successes and enjoyment all began to increase. I remember being delighted with praise from the assistants in the two classes I had for a day and a half respectively as they said I had got the best from the children in such a short space of time.

Meanwhile our social life also took off a little more than it had been – mainly as I now had a clear conscience that I was not 'on the sick'! For example, I enjoyed a school barn dance and we went to a colleague's 50th birthday party with my mother and father. Nick and I had a weekend in Glasgow with Claire and her boyfriend and left Dominic with my parents. We did real 'couple' things again like having drinks in a wine bar and could choose a non-child-friendly restaurant! My confidence in myself was growing at last. I asked Cathy one day to take Dominic to the clinic to be weighed and wrote, 'If my health visitor is there tell her I am fine!' I meant it.

Dominic's second birthday party was at an indoor play place at a craft village. It was busy with other children but I confidently sat amongst the people and chatted to the various friends as the children played. I had enjoyed using the computer to make our own invitations with a scanned photograph of Dominic and once again had returned to the fun of organising an event, even though I did not actually have to do much, except pay! I glowed with pride and love for my two-year-old. Where had my baby gone? As a family we continued at a hectic pace, but we felt that it may make our son sleep at night. In retrospect we did far too much and he wanted to stay awake for the next treat!

In general Dominic did not sleep as well in holiday time as when we were working, maybe due to loss of routine. Back at Cathy's we speculated about his pattern of naps and erratic sleep in general and put it down to all the different things he did each day. She tried to convince me that in time he would sleep. He had erratic spoon skills, a stop/start to toilet training and continued to fight naps and sleep. He liked being busy and learning about his environment. I reassured Cathy that I liked to see his clothes dirty as it showed he had been busy – I was not so paranoid!

During May, Nick was away with school for a week on a residential course with some pupils. I was really proud and relieved that I managed the week's routines without him although I was even more tired. However, the flush of achievement made the adrenaline flow and I survived (with help from my parents). The bond between Nick and Dominic was becoming a little stronger and I liked to watch them do their car cleaning routine together. A wet boy is easier to deal with in the summer. During the half-term holiday we were so organised that Nick even painted the house but I did take Dominic out to stop him being overhelpful. We also chose ourselves a new hall and stairs carpet – a task which would have been impossible the year before. At last we were able to plan and do 'ordinary' things. My pride and affection for Dominic really began to blossom during these months. We had a day out with Margaret, Sue and their children to an ice cream farm and had lunch at a pub. It was one of those occasions which showed my memory gaps as I definitely could not remember having had a school staff Christmas party at the same pub.

At school I continued to cope with all the demands and at my personal development review my boss said she was basically pleased with how I had got on this time. I told Cathy, in Dominic's diary, that I felt she had had a big part to play in this: 'It's so good to know that he is so happy and busy with you and because of that my main worry of being a "working mum" is greatly reduced. Consider yourself appreciated!' The previous night I had been disturbed at 12.30 a.m., 4.30 a.m. and 6 a.m. but I was still smiling. I had begun to manage my time better and if I was tired I would be less strict with myself and rest as opposed to forcing myself to do an unnecessary task. I also had discovered that Dominic loved the new crèche at a local supermarket. This meant I now could shop at the weekend and know he was safe and leave Nick at home to please himself. There was also a café there so I took my grandparents too and we shopped after we had eaten.

Everyone was happy! My grandfather was no longer driving so it was a big help to them. I continued to fit in some exercise classes and managed to win myself ten sessions with a personal trainer at a local gym! This improved my fitness and confidence even more.

Not only was I now back to planning at school, I also had another 'project' to plan for. I used our computer for school work but had also found an internet newsgroup whereby contributors posted information with details of any competitions they had noticed. I had entered many that had been listed, as each night for about half an hour I would relax by entering some of them either by post or e-mail. I had been successful with a few minor prizes but one day I opened an envelope to be informed by a magazine that I had won first prize of a family holiday in Florida! I was so excited! Now I could plan a USA trip. In hindsight it was silly to risk going with the long flights, Dominic's sleep pattern, the worry about his sensitive skin in the sun, etc. plus the additional pressure of whether I would handle it all. It was still early days in my recovery to tackle such a trip but my enthusiasm was so great that Nick did not have the heart to tell me we should not go. I revelled in the prospective joys of the holiday, which we booked for the forthcoming August, and began a new file on where to go and what to do in Orlando.

During the early summer I functioned on a high level of activity and enthusiasm for everything. Maybe the antidepressant pills were now working well in addition to my gratitude and pride at being a working mother again.

Dominic still amazed us all with his excessive energy but he did cause us some concern as the nights were still not good. He was being troubled by itchy skin in spite of all the oils and lotions and was generally bad tempered. He had also been 'under the weather' for a few weeks so I took him to the doctor's. We saw a locum who said Dominic was still congested from a cold, prescribed a decongestant and suggested a different cream for his eczema. His only other support offered was that we should 'just grin and bear it'. It was just as well that I was not as sensitive these days or a comment like that would have upset me deeply. In the months leading up to my hospital stay I would have been distraught at such a simple state-ment, in the way I had reacted to events at my support group. Instead I poured out my woes to Cathy, who replied, 'If you want any time off just let me know! I appreciate he can be very trying at times!' Hence when we broke up for the summer we decided he should carry on going to her for the first week to give us time to rest and prepare for the holiday in America and do some school work. He also spent some time with Nick's mother.

We held a joint birthday barbeque on the first Saturday in August. The sun shone and the garden was full of happy people eating and drinking. We had over 12 adults and eight children, all of whom played well but ours! Dominic sulked and did not like all the other children playing with his toys as they normally were just his. The final straw came when he got hit on the head by a bat, but this actually calmed him down in the end! I did not let the situation upset me and kept busy. It took me ages to actually sit down but when I did I relaxed and congratulated myself on a successful event. A day or two later I had just given Dominic a bath and we were having a toe-biting session on the bed! Although I do look tired both sets of eyes do have a sparkle. I really was getting my life back.

Then we set off for America. The nine-hour flight passed reasonably thanks to a huge bag of tiny toys and activities we had collected in previous weeks to amuse Dominic. Once in Florida the biggest problems were the heat and humidity, which Nick unusually found very oppressive, and the hotel bedroom. It was adequate with two double beds in it and the usual features, but it meant we had no escape from Dominic and were at the mercy of his erratic sleep pattern. The first few days were very taxing for us all. Nick was weary with the heat, Dominic wanted to be permanently on the go and I was overcompensating for them both in my praising and optimism about the holiday. We tended to go out in the mornings for a big American breakfast, shop or sightsee and then head back to the hotel for a midday siesta and lunch. I was terribly concerned about Dominic getting sunburnt so our times in the hotel pool were limited, especially too as he was determined to make for the deep end and bigger children all the time! We would venture out again late in the afternoon then dine in a restaurant. Some evenings went well; others did not either due to the place, our son or both. After the initial few days Nick and I had a heart-to-heart chat about the trip as he was very stressed and disheartened about it all. At home most of our life revolved around this demanding toddler but there were chances for space apart. Here we felt trapped in one room with the responsibility for Dominic's every waking moment. There was no escape. The previous day and night it had been especially hard suiting everyone and if a plane had been available I think we would have got on it.

My continuing optimism saw us through this patch and then we all seemed to settle into the swing of things. We visited many attractions, including Sea World, Disney Marketplace and Gatorland, with a very temperamental toddler in tow, sometimes content and at other times most definitely not. If there was a train, dinosaur, sand or water we were on winning ground. If not, his attention and patience were slim. At the Magic Kingdom we had a tiring but happy day on the rides and walking around. We had a meal with the Disney characters, which we all enjoyed, and were all very impressed by a Lion King show. For me the real magic was the illuminated parade and fireworks when it had gone dark. I remember sitting by a wide-eyed Dominic happily sitting in his buggy watching the floats go by, and suddenly feeling a strong wave of positive emotion. Even Nick looked happy as he attempted to take photographs. The sight of the Magic

Kingdom castle with the fireworks bursting over it is an image seen by many across the world. To actually be there was almost surreal in itself, but as the three of us watched, overcome by the powerful Disney mania, my surge of gratitude to everything and everyone was immense. All the hard work seemed almost worth it for these moments. I felt so proud of myself that amidst all these thousands of people all day I had not had a single panic attack. My only concern had been for the welfare and enjoyment of us all throughout the day. I felt normal. It was sensational.

The final few days in America were much more relaxed, possibly as Dominic had been sleeping through. He and Nick had developed a new routine of 'draw something for me Daddy' and I would have time to please myself, leaving the artists at work. We had learnt to pace ourselves properly and not to expect too much. One day we went to a much quieter park called Silver Springs and had a very relaxing day. As there were no crowds Dominic could run to his heart's content and was a pleasant child. We had not visited any of the water theme parks because we felt we would not be able to appreciate them. However, on our last day we did go to one and all had a terrific time! Typical – we should have gone to more. On our final evening we had a very tasty meal out and back in our room we posed for some family photographs. We had survived and were all still friends! The flight home was fine as Dominic slept for several hours. The in-flight film as we crossed the Atlantic was *Titanic*! Our final verdict was that the trip really was not suitable for a child as young as Dominic. We had only gone as it was a prize and at least we learnt something about the Florida attractions. Maybe one day we shall go again when he is older and we are much wiser! Dominic spent our first few nights back in England with his grandparents to give us some recovery time.

All too soon it was September and we were back to our routine of school and Cathy's again. She observed how much chattier Dominic had become after his holiday so maybe it had benefited him in some way. Evenings at home generally were less fraught. A typical routine was to dine, play in the lounge with a variety of toys (usually trains and dinosaurs), drawing (usually trains and dinosaurs), bath and bedtime story (usually trains and dinosaurs)! This gave me a few hours to do some school work or chores. I still would rarely relax and always had to be busy. I could not just watch television but had to be knitting, sewing or entering competitions at the same time. I continued to keep our weekends very busy and we rarely stayed in without just doing chores. We often did things with my family and often had Sunday dinner at my parents. We had decided that the Golf car was not really big enough for our needs and as we probably would holiday in the UK in coming years (no more hot countries for Dominic yet we thought) then we wanted a bigger car. Nick was thrilled with an estate car and spent hours keeping it in excellent condition. It was my way again of trying to convince him that our life was not too bad. I still felt guilty at times about all the stress he had been put through because of my desire to have a baby.

Luckily the first three days back at school were training and preparation days. At last I had my own class for a full week again and was determined to try my best for everyone involved. My room organising was still important to me and I still spent time on it. I began on the files and information in the areas which were now my responsibility. My team of three classroom assistants and I spent the first few weeks with the children creating plenty of art work. The classroom ceiling resembled an underwater scene with many things suspended. The pupils who often spend time lying on their backs needed to focus on something and this provided a wonderful stimulus and made a huge impact. Everyone in school complimented us on it and I glowed with pride. My planning of the class and new ideas of how to motivate the children began to take off and I buzzed with enthusiasm. I was still tired of course and continued to have some disturbed nights, but generally I coped. Any success would counteract any feelings of inadequacy I felt, giving me the confidence and determination to carry on. My biggest problem was still being in a crowded room. I hated staff meetings and would just sit quietly hoping they would soon finish and dared not actually say anything. In previous years they could not keep me quiet but I had changed. Little by little I did begin to relax and concentrate on the matters in hand. The day I spoke in a meeting was another milestone in my recovery. Likewise, each Friday the classes took it in turn to organise and run assembly. I used to enjoy the 'acting' this involved. Now when it was my turn I was terrified at the prospect of addressing up to 80 people. The first time I just assisted the previous teacher and survived. The next time I had to lead it. My assistants were great as they knew what a challenge it was for me and did all they could to help. My heart was pounding when I began but 20 minutes later when I had successfully presented the assembly I initially burst into tears back in the classroom with the relief of it all. Another major milestone had been achieved. I still was far from confident about it but at least the panic and fear element had subsided.

My achievement at the assembly was magnified even more by receiving a card from one of the parents afterwards. She congratulated me on how well I had looked and thanked me for the support I had given her in the past. I was very touched and really appreciated her gesture. Too often in life we do not tell people how they have helped us – we are quick to complain, but not to compliment. This lady has taught me this lesson and I hope to follow her example.

I began to hold class coffee mornings every half-term to involve the parents of my pupils more and to get to know them. Many of the parents feel isolated as the children are transported to and from school by bus or taxi so we do not have a 'school gate' scenario. I knew how I had begun to appreciate meeting other parents with Dominic and was delighted with the response I got in this instance. However, I confessed to Cathy that I had found the first one to be an ordeal as I was so nervous and feeling unsure of myself. As the months passed a lovely rapport built up between my team and the parents who began to ask when the next one would be. I felt I was able to relate to parents now a great deal more than I used to prior to having a son. I believe I had become much more understanding of pressures they faced. I remember one parent coming to see me as she was having particular problems with her child sleeping at night following an illness. When she told me that she did not feel it was worth her going to bed herself, I asked if she did things like ironing in the early hours. She looked amazed as she confessed that was the case. I had become less judgemental about such problems. Years earlier I would have given her textbook advice about how to get your child to sleep – now I knew it was not that easy. The mother in question said that just the fact that I had genuinely understood her situation was a huge comfort in itself which had made her less tense about it. As professionals, we can be guilty of making people feel inadequate sometimes by offering advice spoken with such apparent knowledge. Occasionally, understanding and empathising can be far more effective and appreciated than purely spouting knowledge.

Another aspect which indicated my return to full health was my final acceptance that a short hairstyle would be good for me! Richard was stunned when I announced 'Just cut it!' and he promptly set to, giving me a sleek, smooth and smart cut. I loved it and began to really take pride in myself again. We met up with Diane and Jon at a pub for a Sunday lunch and to meet their newborn son. Not only did I handle the 'new baby' concept without tears, but Dominic behaved impeccably and kept himself amused with a bag of toys as we chatted and ate.

One evening out which I did find terrifying was when my mother and I went to see the group UB40. There were no seats, just standing. There was also a running bar and people became drunk around us along with suspicious aromas in the air (drugs?). I was scared and clung to a rail in the middle of the theatre. Once the group came on I relaxed a little, but could not wait to leave. I think I would have been apprehensive regardless of my illness though.

Our school Christmas staff night out was much better though. It was a dinner dance followed by a stay in a smart hotel. I wore my wedding dress as people assured me it could easily pass for a white cocktail dress. I felt on top of the world and even a remark that I had come dressed in a nightdress did not dampen my enthusiasm for the night. I drank far too much and danced myself silly but had a wonderful night. Two years previously I had been admitted to a psychiatric hospital – now look at me! Nothing could have dampened my enthusiasm for living that night, not even the wicked hangovers we both had the next day! My brother, wife and son came over for Christmas and we had a pleasant time. I did not cook this year so we went to Nick's family for lunch and on to my family for an evening buffet. Dominic was a joy to watch opening his presents and I again reflected on what huge improvements I had made in two years. On Boxing Day both families came to our house and Dominic and his cousin Brendan became the best of friends, playing contentedly together. Nick and I spent New Year's Eve constructing new shelves for Dominic's playroom. What a sign of the times!

CHAPTER 23

Spreading the word

So the New Year progressed into spring and life was reasonably settled, albeit busy. Although Dominic was proving to be very bright in many areas, the skill needed for toilet training escaped him. Cathy had successfully toilet trained several children and was quite exasperated by his reluctance to even try. He just did not seem to care if he was wet or soiled, but was too busy doing everything else. Again my close involvement with my pupils made me appreciate all his other skills and I felt sure that one day this problem would be solved too. He was just a late developer in this area. Maybe I had learnt to become more relaxed due to my illness and in a way I was pleased that I was not getting worked up about this. Little by little the dry and clean days did come.

In general we were beginning to find life with Dominic to be a little easier. Our morning routine was calm as we prepared everything the night before and we never slept in! After a busy hour at the end of a working day we would sort out the evening meal (chosen and defrosted the night before), put on washing and do other chores. After the meal we could have a relatively peaceful time whilst we watched the news and let Dominic play contentedly on the lounge rug. One programme he still especially enjoyed was watching Jill Dando on *Holiday* – it was so sad when she was murdered. Nick and I would take it in turns to give him a bath later on and read him a bedtime story. Going to bed was never a problem and he went off to sleep quickly.

My love of life and confidence in myself were heightened by more achievements like driving up to see Claire in Scotland with Dominic in our car. Dominic's third birthday celebrations were planned and went well by repeating the same programme as the previous year. I could hardly believe I felt so relaxed. In the Easter holidays we had a rather cold and windy, but successful, holiday in Lanzarote. It was a time-share offer of free accommodation and flights providing you attended a presentation one afternoon. We did this and the remainder of the time enjoyed walks, playing by the pool and meals out together. For once we just stayed at the resort and spent hours just relaxing. We tended to eat out in the early evening when Dominic was at his best and then watch a video back at the apartment. Dominic was distraught one night when a train was blown up! He still had his train fascination. Both he and I were guilty of our moods declining at times – usually because we were hungry. Feed us and we were fine. At least we now had learnt how to 'chill out' together. There was no comparison to the hectic schedules we had set ourselves on other holidays and at home. I had even begun to knit and sew again.

As the summer progressed we all spent productive hours in the garden. Such relaxed times continued to be excellent therapy for us all. Dominic was sleeping better and we coped with the occasional disturbance but these days I was quite happy to have an afternoon or teatime nap if I needed it. The Hanzak pace was busy but calmer during these months and a sunny summer helped. I was also very pleased to be discharged from the psychiatrist who complimented me on my recovery. By now I had stopped all my medication. Gradually I kept forgetting to take it as the need was no longer there. The belief that 'once you start on antidepressants you never stop' did not apply to me. They were merely a form of medication which helped me to cope with life again until I could do so without them. Nick and I asked that if I were to become pregnant again, could the same illness return. Unfortunately the reply was that the probability would be higher second time around. However, as the medical and support services that had helped me this time would be involved right from the birth of a future child, then the chances were it would be controlled or avoided. I was disappointed with the reply, i.e. that it could happen again, and still hoped to conceive one day to 'do it properly', i.e. without the problems. Nick continued to be reluctant.

Our social life was reasonable and we continued to take advantage of offers of help from the grandparents, including overnight stays, either for us to complete school work or just for a break. It was a great relief and very much appreciated. We did have a romantic meal out for our wedding anniversary and concluded that our life was now bearable and a great improvement on the previous years.

Dominic's personality and ability to chatter appropriately was developing fast and consequently the bond between Nick and I with our son was becoming stronger and stronger. He was proving to be a very polite child both at home and outside and he was often complimented for this, which made me feel proud of him.

His independence was growing all the time and he spent increasing sessions contentedly amusing himself in his playroom with his Duplo trains or dinosaurs. Often Dominic would ask Nick for 'a magic carpet story' which he would invent as he went along. It was not just the material items but the little games they invented and played together that warmed my heart.

He was never bored and if he became tired of playing he would chose a video for us to put on for him then sit sucking his thumb, preferably snuggled up to one of us. It made me smile sometimes at the 'pre-mother me' who had vowed she would never let her child watch videos. Oh how I have mellowed!

Generally we managed to balance our school and home lives reasonably well, making time to fit in necessary tasks. At the end of one term I took Dominic into my classroom whilst I sorted a few things out. He had a wonderful time exploring the toys and equipment in the room and I was pleased to get my jobs done. Then we were given the news that the school was in line for a complete OFSTED inspection sometime in the spring. Many of the staff panicked and spent hours worrying and preparing for the visit. Nick and I also spent many hours at school and at home preparing for this and supported and encouraged each other well and refused to let the stress spoil our life. I did have the occasional panic though as I was still battling with trying to find suitable activities for my huge age range of 7–18 year-olds in my class. How was I supposed to meet every criteria the Government guidelines recommended? In special schools we are still required to teach the National Curriculum with modifications. I did my best in the given months and had overcome a problem of recording what the children did in my class by designing and using a picture symbol programme on the computer to create special worksheets which my staff and I completed. It was a way of giving my pupils credit and evidence for any small achievement they may make, e.g. smiling at the feel of something. My worksheets were proving very successful and along with photographs properly labelled, the children had files to be proud of. Of course I got a huge rush of adrenaline about the whole inspection but I seemed to cope with it well. The chief inspector of the OFSTED team interviewed me one day. She explained that the team had been informed of my relatively recent return to work and that they must 'back off' if I was finding the pressure too much. I was grateful for this special dispensation but did not need it. She said that I had been one of the most relaxed members of staff and gave me a very good report. I was honest and informed her that due to my illness I had learnt that the most important thing in life was good health and that having my work looked at did not really bother me. I knew I had a difficult group and if anyone could suggest a better way of planning or delivering the curriculum to my pupils then I would be glad to hear it. I must have been feeling very confident with myself around this time as I read an advert for a deputy headship at a school in the same county and considered myself for it. After giving it some thought, I decided not to apply due to the distance involved. Just considering it was a huge step forward though.

Another great impact on my professional confidence was on a weekend course I attended concerning the teaching of pupils who had profound and multiple learning difficulties. It was wonderful to have the opportunity to converse with other teachers who had similar groups to mine, as often you feel so isolated. The ideas presented inspired me with motivation for the forthcoming years with those children. The course was led by one of the most respected practitioners in our educational area, Flo Longhorn. Many years previously, as a newly qualified teacher, I had been on one of her courses and had been implementing her techniques ever since. We had been invited to take along any files of good practice or ideas to share with other delegates and so I placed one of my pupil's files on the table along with others. I was asked to tell the group about it – another nervous moment, but I succeeded. Afterwards I was invited by the course leader to join her as part of her team on a conference to be held the following year, to run a workshop on my 'innovative' recording techniques! I was thrilled and in coming months she spoke highly of me at other events. With permission, she used some of my pupils' files to include in her book about teaching literacy to such children. Her confidence in me meant a great deal and she continues to motivate me. When she heard about my illness she was even more supportive and has encouraged me to complete this book.

The biggest problem we faced during this period was Cathy's announcement that she and her family were leaving the area in August. We had enrolled Dominic at our local primary school, but it would be over 12 months before he would be full time. Sue could not have him as her children would be attending a school at the other side of town and times would clash. My parents were not retired and Nick's mother lived too far away to take him daily, apart from which we did not feel it was fair on them. I contacted the local social services for a list of child-minders in our area who could take him to the school. The only one on the list who had a vacancy confessed that she did not have much time for the children she minded as she had four of her own. Oh dear. We then discovered that the independent school a few miles away, which my sister had attended for her final years of schooling, took children from the age of three. The fees would be no more than we would have to pay a child-minder, so we went to look around. Dominic was immediately impressed as the nursery teacher gave him a sweet and gold star for chatting to the existing pupils. The added advantage was that a coach could pick him up and drop him off near to the school where we worked and the timing was such that we did not need a child-minder before and after school. Within weeks he had his full school uniform and he began in September.

One physical problem I still had was that whilst I slept I continually had body spasms and seemed to twitch and jerk uncontrollably. Due to this, as a rule Nick and I still tended to sleep in separate rooms as my strong movements would continually wake him up. Normally I would be oblivious to it, but on other occasions I would feel the jerks start in my legs as soon as I relaxed. Consciously trying to keep still made no difference at all. Sometimes, on long journeys, these uncontrolled movements in my legs would start too. Prior to my pregnancy and especially before the ECT I had never experienced this. I wondered if the two were connected. We had put up with this annoying condition for months and in the end I told my GP about it and I was referred to a neurologist. On my suggestion, he investigated possible links between this and any other similar cases reported by people who had been given electric shock treatment. My simple theory was that my body was repeating the 'relax/stimulation/jerking' effect that this treatment had. Was my body somehow recreating this? No link was identified and after a series of tests a cause or cure was not found. Gradually the problem faded, but even now it can happen. Occasionally it is related to me feeling stressed but not always. The other strange phenomenon that now occurs with me is that if I suffer from a side-effect from any new medication, then involuntary body movements will be the symptom. Maybe one day I could be a topic for a student's medical research!

The months passed by. One day I took my grandparents and Dominic to see the aunts in Fleetwood. I reflected on how 'together' I felt on this trip in comparison to similar ones two years earlier. Dominic, my grandfather and I had a walk on the beach and left the ladies, aged between 83 and 94 in the car. Eventually Dominic decided he wanted to go elsewhere and declared that we had better get back to the 'girls'!

We went back to work that September and at the grand old age of 3 years 4 months Dominic started school. I hated it at first as we had some very tearful mornings when the bus arrived. I knew he was fine almost as soon as we were out of sight but the upset stayed with me all day. I remember reading an article about six years being the best age to start school, as they do in some countries. More guilt!

At his next medical review he was seen by a new health visitor. All was well except she criticised us for lifting Dominic out of bed to use the toilet before we went to sleep as she said it was currently not the trend – the reason being that it made the child not used to waking with a full bladder. In view of all our past problems Nick and I felt that if any method worked for us then we used it. Surely this simple two-minute routine was better than having to change a bed in the early hours? The health visitor could not be persuaded otherwise and continued to cast disapproval on us. I felt really angry with her and felt a pang of guilt too as the reaction she caused me to have was probably similar to ones I had made parents feel when I was a well-meaning nursery teacher. I now know that as parents you do what is right for you in the long run. It is good to hear advice but not be criticised when you are trying your best.

Gradually we had learnt that it was not necessary to set ourselves a string of activities at the weekends. Dominic was much more contented to play in his room, leaving us free to do chores, school work or relax. Our pace of life was busy but generally calm. On Sunday 10 October 1999 Dominic and Nick were occupied at home and I decided to go to the local church. Since being back at work my church attendance had been minimal as I did not have either the time or energy. This particular day I had noticed from the local newspaper that the church was holding a special service for World Mental Health Awareness Day. It seemed the right time to go back. I wandered up and was greeted warmly by other parishioners and sat down. The service commenced and we were informed that there were representatives there from the mental health departments and management from the hospital. The vicar spoke of the stigma attached to mental health and recalled some relevant stories. One of the hospital managers also addressed the congregation and agreed by quoting the tale of one of his friends who had lied on a curriculum vitae (CV) and omitted a period of his life when he had been mentally ill. With each word that was spoken, I wanted to shout back that I knew it could be doom and gloom but that I was recovering well. I thought back to the doorway of this very church where I had sat that cold December night in my nightdress; cutting myself with knives; biting my father. I knew the speakers were trying to make the congregation aware of how common mental illness is and how we should all work together to combat the negative aspects, but little by little a wave of appreciation for my recovery and my journey back to the present situation began to overwhelm me. I still am not certain of my religious beliefs but as this wave built in me, I could sense that something or someone was goading me to speak. Such a powerful force began in my toes, worked up my legs, made my stomach tense, my chest expand and my head was fit to burst. I could have sworn that a physical force pushed me to my feet and I suddenly became aware that I was walking up the aisle just before the vicar was about to introduce the next hymn.

People turned to look at me. My heart was racing but I proceeded to ask the vicar if I could tell my story. I stood at the lectern and glanced up. Good grief! What was I doing? I still did not like standing up at school to run a prepared assembly and yet here I was in a church about to make a spontaneous speech! A sea of quizzical faces met mine. I could see my CPN and smiled at his astonished face; I could see a friend of mine and at the back of the church was one of the parents of a child I had taught; familiar faces and strangers. Seeing all these people I felt very nervous and felt my eyes fill with tears, but this strange surge of power I had felt returned and I began to talk. My first few words were broken with the huge lump I had in my throat but once I had started, I relaxed and gave my message. I explained that I had been listening to all the tales and facts this morning but had felt a desire to share my story with everyone there. I admitted that I too had been guilty of judging people badly if they had presented mental illness, but due to my own illness I now understood the condition more. I told them briefly what had happened to me; about the church steps; the psychiatric ward and treatment; the recovery to where I was today as a teacher and mother. I implored them not to make judgements as I had done; that mental illness can and does occur in anyone, not just a supposed 'type'; that you can be treated and that you can recover. I thanked the congregation and vicar for their support, my friends and family, the NHS staff and, as it felt very right at that time, God himself.

With that I walked back to my pew and sat down to applause. I felt flushed and my heart raced even more as the vicar thanked me for being so honest and courageous to tell everyone. A lady sitting near to me squeezed my arm and told me how brave I had been. She had tears in her eyes.

The service proceeded and the surge of feeling I had retracted and was replaced with thoughts such as, 'What the heck did I do that for? What on earth will Nick say?' In a way though, it felt that I had been destined to speak like that. I was, and continue to be, grateful for my recovery and I did want to share it. At the end of the service I was besieged by people. Complete strangers hugged me; the parent I had seen commented that she had wanted to shout that I was a brilliant teacher, but was too shy to do so; my friend complimented me. The Chief Executive of the hospital shook my hand warmly and announced that I had not been 'planted', and in all his years of planning events he could not have hoped for a better representative of the topic. A lady held me and as a tear rolled down her cheek she confessed that she had been taking antidepressants for years, but listening to me had been the best tonic she could have had. After a drink and more positive comments I decided I would go home and report to Nick. Just as I got outside a young lady ran after me. She explained that as part of her job she had been asked to invite users of the 'mental health service' to a conference to be held the next week at the local hospital. She said she had been finding it difficult to find a patient willing to talk about their experiences and as I had spoken this morning she felt I must have been a gift from God to her! I agreed that I would think about it, but I would have to ask permission from school to be excused. We agreed she would speak to me the next day. I excitedly ran home and told Nick what I had been up to.

'Typical!' he said, with a warm smile, 'but well done!'

CHAPTER 24

Making a difference

I was granted a couple of hours away from my class the following Thursday and in the interim I had to prepare a five-minute presentation outlining the factors which had helped or hindered my recovery. There were going to be three other people also giving actual examples of using the mental health facilities in our area. When I had given my impromptu talk at church I had no time to prepare. This time I did and also managed to get myself very worked up and apprehensive! I agonised over what I should wear; should I get changed; my practical classroom outfits were not smart and I would feel scruffy; a suit may look over the top. Poor Nick had to listen to many possible combinations from my wardrobe. In the end I settled for a kilt and black jumper. I had three evenings then to put together a small talk. I did not sleep well as I kept thinking of snippets I should include. By the side of the bed I put a notebook and kept turning the light on to scribble something down which had occurred to me. Part of me was extremely nervous and was cursing myself for agreeing to do it. Another part was very excited by the challenge and the belief that if I could do this, then I was better.

I did several drafts of my small speech and had a few practice runs with my family. I do not think I slept very much the night before. The actual day dawned and I was up early to do my hair and make-up properly. I was useless in class that morning, looking at my watch constantly. Eventually it was time to go and, after plenty of toilet trips, I left school. Just before I left I nipped into Nick's classroom. He came out and gave me a reassuring hug and tried to convince me that it would be fine. I drove to the hospital and was stunned to see a huge white marquee which had been erected adjacent to the rear car park. I did not think it was the venue for the conference as I was only going to address 'a few' staff. I decided to park, doing so with difficulty, and proudly placed a 'Visiting Speaker' note on the dashboard as I had been instructed, to avoid paying the parking fee. I walked in the direction of the marquee and asked someone where the conference was. It was there! Feeling even more worried I wandered inside and Margi, the lady who had asked me to talk, appeared. She explained that it was running late and found me a drink. We sat at the back of the marquee whilst I surveyed the scene. I was amazed how plush it was, complete with chandeliers, proper flooring and festoon curtained sides. At the front was a raised platform with a table and about eight chairs on it. Alongside was a lectern, screen and other presentation paraphernalia. The factor which really struck me was the number of delegates. I counted the number of round tables and estimated there were over 100 people there. Gulp.

The speaker ended his presentation, then everyone had a break. During this time, myself and the other three users or carers were led to the front of the marquee and seated on the top table. I wanted to run! There is nowhere to hide on a top table. Eventually the buzz from the coffee break subsided, delegates took their seats again and the conference proceeded. As other people spoke before me, I had a chance to survey the audience. I could see all the main people who had been involved in my illness scattered about the marquee. My CPN caught my eye and smiled at me, encouragingly. The Chief Executive who had spoken at church did the same. My heart pounded; I kept looking at my prepared talk and was oblivious to the other speakers. Then it was my turn. I took a drink of water from the glass in front of me and made my way to the stand. A technician checked that the microphone was at the correct height and then I had to begin. My years of elocution training suddenly came back as I steadied myself by placing a hand each side of the lectern, took a deep breath and began.

> 'Three years ago I was found outside the local church in the early hours of a December morning wearing just a nightgown. Over the following few days I attacked myself in any way I could find, threw furniture and lost every ounce of logical thought I'd ever had.
>
> Today I am back working as a full-time teacher for a class of children who have profound and multiple learning difficulties; I dote on my three and a half year-old son Dominic, and generally love life with my husband Nick.
>
> So, how did I get to such a state and what helped or hindered me on the way? I hope my personal experiences will help you shape the provision for mental illness in this area.'

So far, so good, but I was rushing. I paused, took another deep breath and continued.

> 'My illness was diagnosed as puerperal psychosis – top of the shop in postnatal depression. I had always longed for children but the latter part of my pregnancy and the birth were complicated and very difficult. At four months old, Dominic had suspected meningitis the week I was due back at work. He was okay but as the weeks went by it became clear to all that I was not. My GP signed me off work with postnatal depression. Three months later I was admitted to the psychiatric hospital and spent almost two months there as an inpatient.'

I was beginning to relax. I kept glancing around the room. There was no sound other than my voice and every eye was on me. Undaunted, I carried on.

'Factors which helped me were:

- *A stay in hospital* – when your usual world is so very threatening you do need escape and refuge to enable you to begin to survive again. Care in the community may have its place but I think sometimes the hospital environment is invaluable.'

I had a quick glance and smiled at one of the lovely nurses who had been on my ward.

- '*A sympathetic GP.*
- *Regular visits from my health visitor, psychiatric nurse and vicar* – being listened to and reminded that you are not a failure, but ill, took me a long time to accept.'

Another smile for my vicar's wife, also a cleric, who was there as part of her role as hospital chaplain.

- '*Gradual discharge* from everything – appointments, medication, etc. – this enables you to build up your confidence in the world again.
- *ECT* – the relaxation for the few moments whilst the anaesthetic took effect were sheer heaven at the time, and maybe this treatment did help me turn the corner back to recovery.
- *Looking backwards* – on very bad days it helped to be reminded of small improvements I had made rather than dwelling on the things I could not do, e.g. last Tuesday you would not answer the phone; this Tuesday you picked it up and said "hello". A small step maybe, but positive.
- *Physiotherapy and occupational therapy* – spending time going through relaxation techniques and finding me therapeutic activities. I had never found this a problem before my illness but I had lost all concept of this. Even today I find myself concentrating on breathing exercises in times of stress and picture a flickering candle.
- Opportunities to *exercise*.
- *Time* – the great healer.
- A supportive *family and friends*.'

Hey! This was going well. I was actually enjoying myself. I was speaking to a large audience. Was this for real?

'Factors which did not help:

- Drastic *changes in medication* and uncertainty of what I should be on.
- *Unsympathetic staff* – for example, being told off for knocking a vase over when my body was out of my control due to a medication change.
- A *support group* – useful in some ways, but I learnt the best way to cut my wrists listening to a story told by another sufferer there.
- *Overpowering consultations* – at my worst in hospital I went in to see the doctor and was faced with about eight professionals – very scary when talking to one person is such an ordeal.
- Putting Dominic on the *at risk register* – put in front of a panel as a family just added more strain to us all.'

Quick look at social worker.

- *'Pressure from work* to return or lose my job.
- *Being told 'You look well'* – you might do but inside you are a wreck. A comment such as 'Your hair looks nice today' is much better.
- *After-care* – on the whole it has been good, but I do appear to have developed involuntary spasms when I sleep since my illness and yet I now have to wait for months to be seen by a neurologist to even begin to investigate the problem.

My additional suggestions:

- *More alternative remedies*, e.g. St John's Wort, homeopathic approaches, massage.
- *Assertiveness training and stress management techniques* – we are told to say 'No' to strangers as a child, but many of us are not good at saying it to adults as we grow up.
- *Inpatient care with a flexible approach*, e.g. being allowed to sit with staff in the night is much more beneficial than lying painfully awake for hours after being sent to bed.
- More *support for the direct family* and *information for employers*.

I am very grateful to the local National Health Service for all the support and services they provided which have enabled me to make such a good recovery.

I wish you continuing success with all your patients and hope my contribution today has been useful.'

I had done it! There was a burst of loud applause and as I smiled and picked up my papers I noticed a few people wiping their eyes. I had done it!

It felt great! I wanted to punch the air. I wanted to hug everyone. I wanted Nick to have been there and share the pride and elation I was feeling. I had actually done it! I returned to my seat on the top table as a different woman. All my confidence which had been sapped from me over the last few years had come back like a tidal wave. I was on top of the world and could not stop grinning (like a mad woman!). In typical conference style, after the short talks given by the users of the service, each table then had to discuss and work together on a sheet of relevant questions looking at improvements. Some of the executives came to chat to us as we huddled together in an area at the side of the top table. Nothing stopped me now and hardly anyone else got a word in as I added my thoughts on the questions raised.

Then it was a break for lunch. I decided I may as well stay and headed off towards the queue. My CPN came over to me and congratulated me on my talk. He was amazed that I had been able to do it now on two occasions and he confessed that he could not address a crowd like that and he had not been ill. He said he was really pleased for me and added that I had also done his reputation a favour. Other people came to say they had been impressed by my words. Then a middle-aged lady approached me, her eyes filled with tears. She warmly held me by the shoulders and said that she had worked in the mental health field for many years, but in recent years her own teenage son had suffered a breakdown. Most days she said she despaired that she would ever get her 'old' son back, but listening to me had filled her with so much hope that one day it would happen and she could not thank me enough for that. I felt emotional too. She stressed to me that I should write a book about my illness and recovery as it would help so many people. Although my problems were connected to the birth of my son, my symptoms and experiences related to so many mental health issues that it would help across the whole spectrum.

I would have liked to chat to this lady more, but we were interrupted by a lively lady with a camera who asked for my photograph as a record of the day.

'We must have the star,' she said.

I know I smiled for those photographs! Apparently it is still displayed in a collage in the new mental health unit of our hospital, but I have never seen it. I returned to school on a definite high and remained so for a long time.

Two days later I began to write this book. I collected together all the diaries and notes I had made over the period and started to collate them on the computer. The first weekend I wore myself out and made myself tired for work. I realised I would have to balance this project with everything else and only do it when I had time and energy. I knew I could not work to a deadline as that would cause me unproductive stress.

Meanwhile our family and working lives ticked over. At school I had a greater confidence with my class and enjoyed seeing my pupils achieve even the smallest of steps. I used my own experiences in dealing with their parents and liked the camaraderie between the staff in my area. One of my classroom assistants said I was 'nice to be with' after her husband had a terrible accident and subsequent traumas. She said I seemed to have a real understanding of what it was like to suffer and would listen and be genuinely sympathetic without being patronising. I was very grateful for such a comment.

We had a good Millennium Christmas and New Year at home. My brother and all his family came over from Zimbabwe and, whilst here, they sorted out jobs, schools and a new home near Oxford. My parents, Kevin and Annie, had tickets to go to the Dome for the Millennium night, so we had a tasty meal at home and tried to spot them on television. I think Dominic was waiting for a full head and shoulders shot of his grandmother, instead of the Queen! We saw the New Year in with fireworks and champagne and again felt very grateful for our current lifestyle.

Dominic continued to do well at school apart from the occasional toilet mishap! It felt weird going to his parents' evening and being 'on the other side'. His teacher assured us that he was a bright boy who always finished first and did the task properly. He was determined, affectionate, liked to make people laugh, had an excellent vocabulary, was very active and alert and kind hearted. He was the only child in his class of 20 to have a special sticker for having a gold star on every page of his writing book. We were very proud of him. We felt too that the older children on the coach had made him more confident and sociable than other children his age. As they had trendy radio stations on the coach journey, Dominic also had better pop music knowledge than we did! He continued his cute ways of endearing himself to us and for Mothering Sunday recited the verse in the card he had made me:

'You can squeeze bananas,
you can squeeze ripe plums,
but when you're feeling sad,
it's good to squeeze your Mum!'

He also tried to make his own version about Dads!

Towards the end of January I was invited by the local Director of Nursing and Patient Services, Mandie, to participate as a speaker at a national nursing conference to be held in London that November. She was involved on the planning committee for the conference and they wanted a patient who had recent experiences of the healthcare system to address the delegates and my name had sprung to mind. She had heard me speak in the marquee and said that my 'eloquent and often moving' description of my experiences had encouraged the NHS trust to engage the users of the services in future planning and development. The national conference was entitled 'Making a Difference' and was to address 'essence of care' clinical benchmarks to be introduced in hospitals for nursing care. My talk would 'set the scene'.

I was very flattered and decided that I would like to be involved. My head teacher gave me leave of absence for the date and supply cover would be arranged. I then had almost nine months to prepare. I bought two suits and a jacket in the sales as possible outfits, but my mother treated me to a smart dress and waistcoat nearer the time. I also had these months to work out what I would say. As the planning got underway it appeared that I would follow a Member of Parliament and my half-hour talk was to be the keynote presentation for around 500 nurses! Now look at the trouble I had let myself in for! I admit that I probably became a bore about this event and it dominated my thoughts. Mandie gave me the information about the main benchmark areas and I planned my experiences around them. I decided that I would actually write it during part of the school summer holidays. My parents took Dominic and his cousin for a fun-filled visit to London, so that I could be left in peace.

In the interim, I had more direct involvement with the NHS. My grandfather had been diagnosed as having lung cancer. He had been a barber and sold cigarettes which became part of his life. I remember hearing his cough as a child and combined with my parents' dislike of smoking it was a habit that had never interested me. He had managed to live until 89 and used to say he had been given a 'good innings', but the suffering he went through the last days of his life were horrendous. For months it had been obvious he was not well but he tried to hide his pain from us all and seemed determined to stay at home with my grandmother. He had nurses visiting at home and it was they who sent for an ambulance one day, as he could not get his breath. Unless you have had experience of a close family member in hospital, I do not think you realise how it takes over everything for the rest of the family. All usual routines are dismissed and phone calls revolve around the patient and visiting times. It is very tiring and stressful for all concerned. Unfortunately Nick had to go away with a class from school for a week, but I managed to handle the hospital visiting and our usual routines.

The side ward my grandfather was in, had another five elderly men suffering with lung problems. The wheezing and coughing were awful to listen to. My grandfather's pain increased and he was put on high levels of pain relief. In the middle of one night, my parents were sent for as he was hallucinating and had become violent due to the drugs and the staff were unable to intervene due to hospital policy. My parents found him in a side room, ranting and raving about rats running around. He calmed down eventually and then he seemed to plateau for a week or two. During this time, he was happy and content despite his pain. I even took Dominic in to visit, but always took some paper and pens to amuse him. Another of the patients took a shine to Dominic, who was well behaved, and one day called him over and gave him a pound coin as a treat. A few days later, as we were going into the hospital, we passed a man who looked very similar to this gentleman, but he was obviously up and dressed. Dominic noticed him and, thinking it was the 'ill' man, brightly said, 'Oh, I'm so glad you're feeling better. Are you going home?'

Sadly, the actual kind man had died. One day my grandfather commented to me that he had had a good day – his bed was comfortable, he had had some good conversations and his apple pie was lovely. He had always enjoyed company and the chat between him and his fellow patients must have been similar to those he had enjoyed as a barber. I felt grateful to the hospital for giving this to him. However, as a family we felt that sometimes nurses did not give my grandparents the respect they deserved, as elderly people. One nurse was particularly impatient with them both when they were asked if they wanted a drink. Their hesitant reply resulted in the young nurse being abrupt and rude with them whilst she chewed her chewing gum with greater force. No matter how pressured a job is on the wards, surely courtesy and patience should still be paramount?

One afternoon my mother, grandmother and I were invited to attend a case conference about him. My 90-year-old grandmother was very distressed by the procedure as there must have been at least ten professionals involved in the meeting. I really felt for her and it reminded me of the meeting I had to go into when in the psychiatric ward. When you feel so vulnerable and worried, a sea of well-meaning but daunting professionals is too much. Basically the consultants had decided that there was no more the hospital could do and that my grandfather should be transferred to the local hospice for palliative care. We did not dispute this fact, but felt it was unnecessary for it to be done in this way. All my grandmother needed was one person informing her of this. One of the nurses suggested that we would be able to take him out occasionally, maybe home for a meal. I resented this approach. He was 89, suffering badly, with death coming as a welcome relief. I did not want false hopes. I wanted his pain to end.

A few days later he was transferred to the hospice and had a pleasant room, sponsored by Marks and Spencer. We joked that this was appropriate as he had sat on their seats many a time waiting for my grandmother to shop 'round the food'. By this stage, though, he was unconscious. The staff that tended him were wonderful. They asked about what he had been like before his illness and made his last few days as bearable as possible. It was obvious that he would not be with us for much longer and I appreciated being granted a day off school to be with him and my family. My parents and I went that morning. He was a tiny figure in the bed and we were shocked by how laboured his breaths were. The pain-relief mechanism was hidden and he had no outward signs of tubes or medical intervention. The staff nurse tactfully and sensitively told us that 'it would not be long' and left us alone. We decided that my parents would go and bring my grandmother and I would stay. Up to this period in my life I had been very lucky not to lose anyone close to me. Death was something that I had not really dealt with before now. I sat close to him, held his hand and chattered away. I remembered one of my colleagues had told me that she had seen her mother die of cancer and reached this point of wishing her suffering to end. She confessed that she had told her to go and shortly afterwards she had died. I felt like that now so I told him that we would take him back to his home town to be buried. I described the journey we would take and said I would ask that the hearse drive past his beloved barber's shop. At this his breathing changed and he seemed to utter a sound. I reassured him that we would all take good care of my grandmother but now it was time for him to go. I thanked him for all the good and not so good times we had shared and told him I loved him.

Almost on cue, it seemed, two nurses came in and suggested I left whilst they gave him a wash and made him more comfortable. I sat in the deserted lounge and just thought of all the times we had spent together. In days gone by he had been the typical 'life and soul' of any party; he was sociable, humorous, hardworking and popular with all who knew him. My grandfather also had a stubborn streak and could be short tempered but he was always good to me. I remembered him sitting on his convector heater in the shop when he was between customers. I remembered the way he used to jingle coins in his pockets as he talked. I remembered his many tales, often using the expression 'any road' instead of 'well'. I remembered him crawling around the floor with Claire on his back pretending he was a horse. I remembered him pushing Dominic's pram along the seafront. I remembered.

A nurse came to tell me that they had finished and just as I got to his door, my parents and grandmother appeared. She gasped at how ill he looked and sobbed into my mother's shoulder, saying that she did not realise how bad he was. I held his hand as he appeared to mutter something (my father said it was 'Where the heck have you lot been?') and he began to sit up momentarily as I held his hand again. He flopped back down, took a few deep breaths and was gone.

The nurse checked his pulse and gently said that he was now at peace and not suffering any more. Her colleague appeared too and said that they regretted they had not been able to get to know him a little. He would have liked them. All of us cried and, in true British style, a cup of tea was brought. Meanwhile one of the nurses nipped a flower from the vase and placed it by my grandfather's pillow. I kept hold of his hand and was amazed how quickly it went icily cold. We stayed with him for several hours, just chatting. My grandmother kept talking to her late husband and declared, 'I'll say one thing – you've not left me with a rubbish family!'

She is always at her strongest in troubled times.

The funeral was held the following week. The church was quite full and many of my grandfather's customers and neighbours were there. The service was a suitable memorial of his life and then we followed the hearse along the diverted route past his former shop, and on to the cemetery where we left him surrounded by the sea breeze he loved.

Meanwhile the rest of our lives ticked over. Dominic celebrated his fourth birthday which we held at home. His favourite part was helping me make a dinosaur cake. The planning, preparing, running and aftermath made us decide we would go to a venue for future ones! I had continued entering competitions on the internet and was stunned to win £5000 from a site! The only problem was that when we discussed what we should do with it we decided it was nowhere near enough! After various debates we settled on having a new kitchen installed which we all would benefit from. We had a wet summer holiday in a converted byre in Devon but at least enjoyed being a family together. By the end of the summer my London talk was complete and after several meetings with Mandie to edit small parts, it was ready – and so was I.

CHAPTER 25

And so to London

My excitement about the talk I was preparing to give in London was further fuelled by letters from Mandie, from the organisers and seeing my name in print in all the conference advertisements in the main nursing press. I stood in a supermarket one day and looked through one of the relevant journals and found it. I wanted to dig the person next to me and say 'That's me!' I refrained but I admit I was so pleased about it. I thanked Mandie for thinking of me in the first place and helping to restore a huge chunk of confidence which had left me for so long. I had inflicted my talk on my family and some colleagues at school as rehearsals. Letters and e-mails between myself and the conference organisers continued so we could check details, e.g. that I needed to use a slide projector. I had decided that my talk would be more effective if I added some relevant family photographs for people to relate to. The conference organisers suggested I booked my own travel tickets and they would refund it after the event. One evening I found a suitable train and booked the cheapest fare. I would travel down the afternoon before and return in the evening the next day. I would have the afternoon to spend in London as I chose. I looked up details of the hotel in Kensington where I would stay for the night and also details of the conference venue. I had practised my make-up, got several different pairs of tights to try and treated myself to new nail polish. I gave my new dress and waistcoat a stroke every time I opened the wardrobe.

The night before I was due to go to London I packed and double-checked everything countless times and just before I went to bed checked my e-mails. I could hardly believe my eyes when I read one from the Lionel Richie fan club. I am a member as he is my all-time favourite singer. He was due to be a guest at an afternoon chat show in London on the very afternoon I had to spare! They were inviting fans to be part of the audience and to do so you had to send an e-mail to the appropriate person. This had to be fate! My childish level of excitement for the talk was now added to by the prospect of meeting my 'hero'! A few years previously, my mother and I had been to one of his concerts and waited at the stage door for hours after, just to see him for a few moments. This chance could not be missed so I replied, giving my mobile phone number and the hotel number as successful applicants would be contacted. I did not sleep well that night, surprise, surprise.

Once in London I found myself a taxi and checked into the hotel a little while later. My room was small but very modern with chic white linen and pale wooden furniture. On the dressing table was a bottle of champagne and a note which read 'Well done, love, we're very proud of you, Mum and Dad'. I beamed and immediately phoned them and Nick to report I had arrived safely. I had given up on the Lionel Richie event as I had not heard anything. I unpacked and wandered downstairs to enquire if Mandie had arrived. Her train had been delayed so I went back to my room and flicked the television channels. My mobile phone rang and it was the television company giving me details of how to be in the audience for the show tomorrow. Yes! All I had to do was get across London the following afternoon when my talk had been given! When Mandie arrived she was as excited for me as I was. We are both around the same age and have the same taste in music. We opened the champagne and drank it whilst we chatted until late and generally had a very pleasant couple of hours.

I did not sleep, for fear of not waking up in time. I had set the alarm in the room but did not trust it. I wished I had told Nick to phone me just in case. I made myself several hot drinks and just could not settle for a weird mixture of fear and excitement. Of course I was sleeping blissfully when the alarm did go off and the reality of the day dawned on me. I was going to talk to 500 people. I showered, dressed, put on my make-up in the hope of disguising the bags I felt under my bleary eyes and made my way downstairs to meet Mandie at the arranged time. I felt sick. For some reason I was conscious of every part of my body. My feet felt like stone in my boots; my tights felt like they were suffocating me; my new dress was like a corset. I felt that everyone was looking at me. Mandie introduced me to many people involved in the conference who were also staying at the same hotel. She was very talkative. I was not. I hardly ate anything. I wanted to go. I do not know where. Just go. She assured me that she always got nervous before giving a presentation, but she said I would be fine. Often she had reminded me that my audience were primarily nurses and thus essentially caring people. Even those who were now executives at high levels had all started out on the wards. They were not aggressive business people who were seeking personal gains, just genuine, caring people. I went back to my room, brushed my teeth again and packed up. Yes, my papers and slides were still there. I spoke to Nick and Dominic on the phone, then my parents. How I wished they could have been there cheering me on. They reassured me that they would be thinking of me and I met up with Mandie again.

It was a beautiful winter morning, cold and crisp but very sunny. Once again I felt all my senses heighten as we turned into a bustling Kensington High Street en route to the venue close by. The traffic, the buses, the pedestrians, the shops, all seemed bright and noisy. We soon came to the conference centre and I was warmly greeted by a couple of the staff I had communicated with. There was a general mêlée of delegates queuing up to register and collect their packs. Mandie and I were ushered up to the quiet speakers' room where drinks were being served. I was introduced to a number of people from the top ranks of British nursing and made to feel very welcome. I began to relax a little, especially as Mandie kept telling everyone that I had a date with Lionel that afternoon! I had been told to think up a question to ask him and every now and then she came up with a suggestion. At least it made me relax a little. I was given a name badge and we duly went down to the auditorium. It seemed huge and dark. It was all navy blue – seats, walls and tiered floor. The stage and screen seemed enormous. It reminded me of the cinemas before multi-screens were introduced, as it was so big. A helpful young man took my slides and showed me how to operate the projector. He tested one and I was stunned to see a 20 foot version of myself!

Luckily the speakers did not have to sit on the platform but on reserved seats in the front row. This was kinder and less stressful. A few well-presented and efficient lady speakers opened the conference and outlined the importance of the benchmarking initiative. Unfortunately there were problems on the underground that morning and some delegates were late. During the first couple of hours there was a steady stream of latecomers and eventually the hall was filled to capacity. As my slot approached I tried to keep as calm as possible and kept my breathing slow, picturing that flickering candle. I knew I would get through this and would be so happy to do so. The thought of my feelings afterwards was the driving force that gave me confidence to take my place on the stage and deliver my long-awaited presentation. With a deep breath and a final check of the microphone, I began my talk, entitled 'What Matters To Patients'.

'Good morning ladies and gentlemen,

This is my son Dominic and I at our local church on his christening day about four years ago [see Figure 1]. A few weeks later I was found on these steps in the early hours of a December morning wearing just my nightdress. Over the following few days I attacked myself and my family in any way I could find and lost every ounce of logical thought I'd ever had.

Today I am back working as a full-time teacher for a class of children who have profound and multiple learning difficulties; I dote on Dominic who is a bright, happy and affectionate child, and generally love life with my husband Nick. This was taken on our wedding day in 1995 [see Figure 2].

My illness was diagnosed as puerperal psychosis – the most severe form of postnatal depression. I had always longed for children but the latter part of my pregnancy and the birth were complicated and very difficult. Our new baby Dominic did not sleep

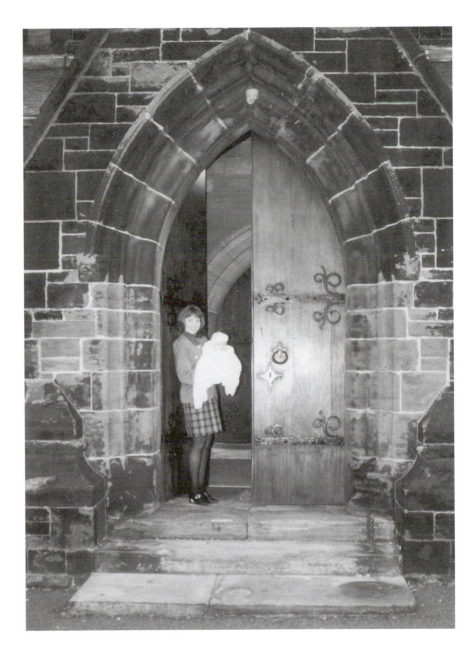

Figure 1   Dominic and I at the church doorway on his christening day

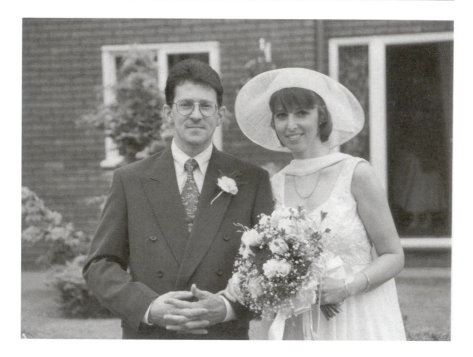

Figure 2   Nick and I on our wedding day

well and at four months old he had suspected meningitis the week I was due back at work. He recovered but as the weeks went by it became clear to all that I was not well. Normally I am a very organised, busy person who copes with life well. However, I began to feel I was losing control of everything. I withdrew from all my family and friends. I became increasingly housebound and would not even answer the telephone. Poor Nick never knew what to expect each evening on return from work – a smiling wife who had made a meal or a rambling wreck in her dressing gown bemoaning that he should feed himself. The week before Dominic's first Christmas I totally broke down, as I have described, and was admitted to the local psychiatric hospital, spending almost two months there as an inpatient and many months as an outpatient.

It has been a comparatively long road back to recovery but obviously something has helped me to be able to speak to you all here today. In addition to the nursing experiences associated with my pregnancy and son, earlier this year I witnessed geriatric and cancer care with the death of my grandfather. Through all of these periods I have been on the receiving end of many aspects of nursing, some of which have definitely aided recovery and unfortunately some which have not.

During my talk today I shall base my anecdotes, where appropriate, around the areas outlined in the Benchmarking Initiative. Obviously my comments are purely a personal account of what matters to patients, but I hope I also speak for many others and consequently will help you shape and improve aspects of patient care in the UK.

Primarily I do feel qualified to comment upon the 'safety of patients with mental health needs'. Initially, in dealing with mental illness we all need to remember it *is* an illness – my psychiatric nurse would be proud to hear me say that as he spent weeks convincing me that this was the case when at the time I put it down to my failures. So many people told me that I 'wasn't the type' to get postnatal depression and I believed them.

With the absence of physical scars or injury it is often hard to realise that a person is suffering. For example, in this photograph

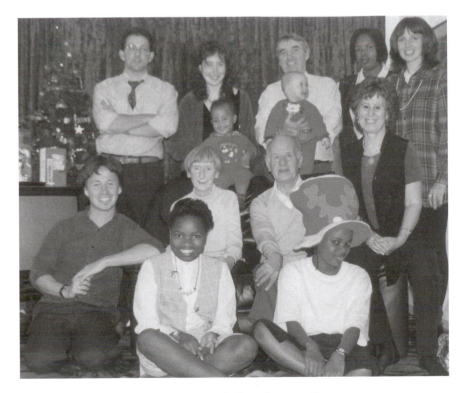

Figure 3   My family, taken on Dominic's first Christmas Day

[see Figure 3] taken on Christmas Day when I had been allowed out from the psychiatric ward, you could say I look fine. In reality I had just been discovered shaking Dominic, which led to him being placed on the Child Protection Register. Likewise, if you look closely my fingers are in plasters from me gouging holes in them and my wrists bandaged from cutting myself with a photograph frame.

Remember that *real* understanding is needed by all involved. Do not judge a mentally ill person just as you would not judge someone with a bacterial infection or heart problem. At times I felt that certain nursing staff were very impatient in the psychiatric ward, especially with some of the elderly ladies. Matters that normally are of little importance can seem colossal when you are mentally ill. For example, imagine how you have felt in a sudden crisis, such as losing the sight of your toddler in a busy shop. Your heart pounds, you can't think straight and you feel that they are gone forever. Now imagine that same feeling of panic, and you are only having to sit in a day room with a few people, yet those same symptoms have made you freeze to the spot. How would you like to be grabbed by the arm, told to stop being silly and pushed into a chair? Please remember that to them it is a very real fear that needs a great deal of patience and understanding.

I could never appreciate before my illness how people felt with apparently irrational fears of lifts, escalators or even spiders. These days I now can empathise with people's fears and worries. I try some of the same techniques with them which have helped me face the human race again. Help sufferers to aim for little steps of progression, be positive, telling them that they can do it and that they are alright, that the challenge will soon be over and imagine how proud they will feel when they have done it – like I will be by 10.30 today!

This is one of my favourite 'feeling better' photographs [see Figure 4]. I had just had my hair cut, I had lost some weight and we had just had lunch out with a friend who had had a baby. I'd coped with it all and was thrilled as it was all a big achievement at the time.

Keeping a mentally ill person safe hopefully means a stay in hospital. When your usual world is so very threatening, you do need escape and refuge to enable you to begin to survive again. Care in the community may have its place but I think sometimes the hospital environment is invaluable. I found the proximity of other patients in the ward to be a great comfort in my early days in hospital. A room on my own would have been horrific initially

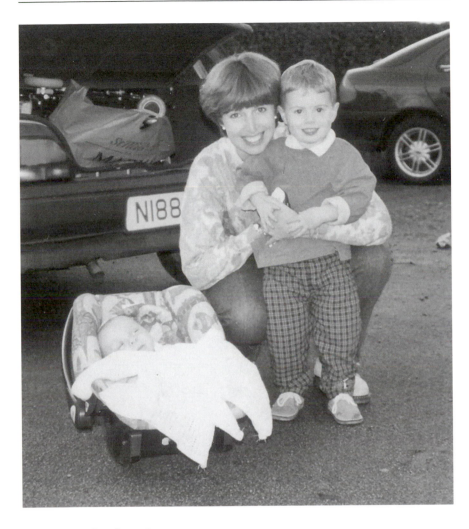

Figure 4   Feeling better!

as the person I was most scared of was myself. Individual rooms may not always be best.

Please try to consider inpatient care with a flexible approach. For example, being allowed to sit with staff in the night is much more beneficial than lying painfully awake for hours. One night I was very distressed and attacked myself and the staff who came to aid me. Eventually when I dissolved into tears they wrapped me in a blanket, gave me a milky drink and let me just sit with them whilst they chatted on night duty. Those few hours set me back on the road to recovery. Being left in the darkness again would probably have made me worse and led to more harmful behaviour.

Another technique I found helpful was stepped and paced approaches, such as your bed position in a ward, gradual discharge from appointments and medication. It enables you to build up your confidence in the world again and be safer within it. Conversely, drastic changes were damaging, especially in medication as the side-effects were very frightening at times.

The most negative aspect of my hospital stay was an unsympathetic member of staff. For example, I was reprimanded and told I was a nuisance for knocking a vase over when my body was out of my control due to a medication change. The following night they found me hiding in a dark corner, hurting myself again, because I was too scared to ask the staff for help.

In general I feel that more support for the direct family and information for employers would be very helpful for all involved. Mental illness is an area that still needs a great deal of public education for sufferers to be helped. If I had needed major surgery an official sickness leave would have been given and accepted by everyone. The same boundaries are not set for mental illness and the pressure to return to work makes it much harder for the patient and difficult for employers to plan around.

Another benchmarking standard which is obviously important to patients is 'privacy and dignity'. I found these aspects especially relevant to my grandfather's treatment. Here he is with me on my wedding morning [see Figure 5]. Unfortunately some younger nurses did not treat him and my grandmother with the respect they deserved; for example, tutting at their hesitant reply to being asked if they wanted a drink. Chewing gum, huffing, puffing and generally appearing to be bad tempered are not good nursing qualities and do not help any patient. I am well aware that people can be annoying but they should not be admitted to hospital for care and basically be insulted. However, most of the time staff were very kind to him and made his last weeks of life as happy as possible.

I feel that long visiting hours are not conducive to privacy or dignity – as a visitor on my grandfather's ward I often felt intrusive upon other patients. For the visiting families it can put extra pressure and stress to have to stay. As a patient it can be exhausting trying to make small talk and also other people's visitors can drive you demented with noise.

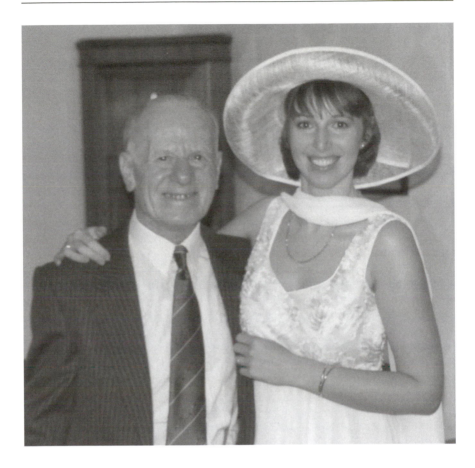

Figure 5   My grandfather and I

Not all of us can look this cute in a nappy [see Figure 6] and 'continence' is a vital part of hospital care and rightly recognised as another area to be checked. As humans we like to feel clean and comfortable and as it is often the most vulnerable who have this problem it must always be dealt with tactfully, sensitively and discreetly. For those whom incontinence is a new problem this must be upheld even more. It caused my grandfather a great deal of distress in his final weeks and we were all grateful to staff who were sensitive to this.

Likewise, when I awoke in the night following emergency surgery after giving birth to Dominic, I had tubes coming from everywhere it seemed [see Figure 7]. I was in a room by myself,

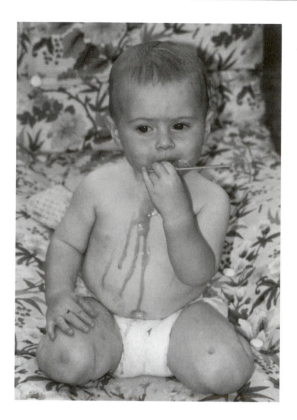

Figure 6   Looking cute in a nappy!

with dimmed lighting and just my newborn son. Every hour or so the same nurse came to clean me up and change the bedding due to my considerable discharges. It is the nearest I have been to being incontinent but that nurse was wonderful in dealing with me – she explained what she was going to do then chatted to me about many things as she efficiently sorted me out. She made me feel like a pampered child and not a disgusting smelly creature.

Always remember that although incontinence may be something you deal with every working day, to the patient it may not be and they need genuine compassion to deal with it.

I agree that 'record keeping' is compulsory and is very useful, but it has to be correct and passed on! Many aspects of my pregnancy were not followed properly because someone had not passed on the necessary notes or information. My treatment for urinary tract infections at seven months seemed erratic because I was never

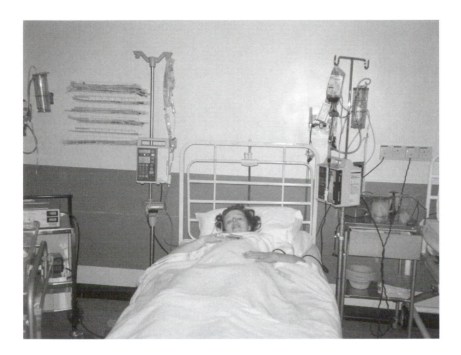

Figure 7   Not at my best

seen by the same doctor twice, each relying on the previous notes. The named consultant at the time never came to see me during my 10-day stay. Later, my new consultant did not know about my problematic delivery and subsequent surgery until my six-week check-up. No one had told her and to this day I have never been given a full explanation of all the complications involved, the reasons for it and if it could happen again.

One night in the psychiatric ward I was suffering badly from a different drug. It was giving me whole-body spasms which I could not control. I tried to relax but could not, then eventually wandered about and hurt my face on a bookshelf when I collided with it. I recalled the events to Nick the next day to try to convince them to do something to help me. No record had been made of my appalling night and I felt betrayed by everyone.

Dominic has begun to show interest in 'food and nutrition'. Here he is making his birthday cake [see Figure 8]. I liked my food in the three hospitals I stayed in! We were given several choices of what and how much we wanted. Generally the quality was good;

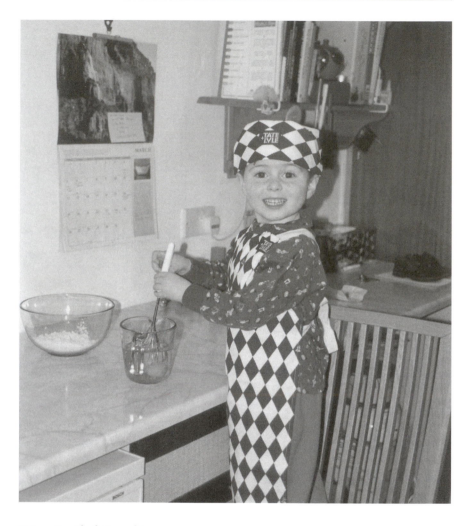

Figure 8 Chef at work!

healthy but comforting. It tasted fresh and not stewed up. Crockery is much better than plastic alternatives. I appreciate that the use of plastic cups is safer and more hygienic, but you still cannot beat a drink from a proper cup. Please can we have them!

Drink time in hospital can be a treat to look forward to, but why, oh why do you have to wake patients up at the crack of dawn with one when it is hours until breakfast? After almost a year of never having more than two to three hours of undisturbed sleep at any time, imagine my exasperation at being woken up for a grotty cup of tea at 7 a.m. and being told off for being lazy!

A few days before my grandfather died I asked how his day had been on the ward. He replied 'Ee love, a day good enough to go in a scrap book – I've had some good conversations, people have been kind to me, my bed's comfy and I had a lovely piece of apple pie for my dinner!' That's what mattered to him.

Another area I agree is important for all patients, no matter what their illness is, has to be 'hygiene and mouth care'. My grandfather was very grateful to be shaved and changed into clean pyjamas, even the day before he died. All patients feel better if helped to be kept clean. A bath and having body lotion on can be very thera-peutic. Even a bed bath and having your teeth cleaned can be the highlight of your morning when in hospital, or if being nursed at home, and its power should not be underestimated or the process rushed. For the visiting families it is also a relief to see that your loved one has been cared for, and it is greatly appreciated.

I think hospitals should encourage appropriately trained staff to give manicures and hairdressing to patients. It would help patients relax, feel pampered and sleep better – just like this [see Figure 9]. Maybe visitors could buy vouchers for such treatments instead of grapes, chocolates and flowers.

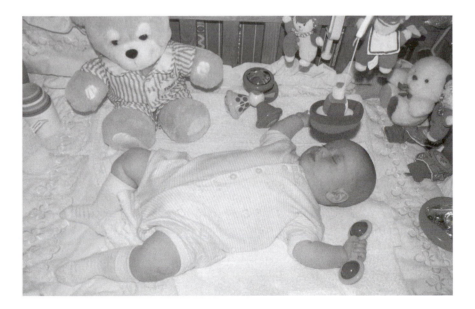

Figure 9 Sleeping like a baby

Everyone likes to be complimented on their appearance but as a psychiatric patient I never found comments such as 'You look better today' or 'You're looking well' to be positive. Indeed, you might appear so but inside you are a wreck and such comments just add to your guilt that you do not look ill so you mustn't be. A compliment such as, 'Your hair looks nice today' is much better.

I was pleased to see 'principles of self-care' listed as one of the new standards as I believe they have helped me enormously. For example:

1   Physiotherapists and occupational therapists spent time going through relaxation techniques and finding me therapeutic activities. I had never found this a problem before my illness but I had lost all concept of this. Even today I find myself concentrating on breathing exercises in times of stress and picture a flickering candle.

2   Looking backwards. On very bad days it helped to be reminded of small improvements I had made rather than dwelling on the things I could not do, e.g. 'Last Tuesday you would not see any visitors but today you've seen two.' A small step maybe, but positive.

3   Regular meetings with my GP, health visitor, psychiatric nurse and vicar. Being listened to and reminded that you are not a failure, but ill, took me a long time to accept. If you learn to open up and talk to professionals in dealing with your difficulties then as you become better you learn to handle them yourself.

4   Opportunities to exercise are important even if just a walk down the ward or visit to the hospital occupational therapy department or gym. It was a great feeling to begin to feel the adrenaline buzz after being stagnant for so long and one I have continued to return to. I even managed to climb up Snowdon [see Figure 10].

5   A support group for postnatal depression sufferers was useful in some ways, such as sharing ways of coping strategies, e.g. assertiveness training and stress management techniques. We are told to say 'No' to strangers as a child, but many of us are not good at saying it to adults as we grow up. However, such groups need careful monitoring as I also learnt there the best way to cut my wrists listening to a story another sufferer told. I sometimes felt that the system did not suit everyone and, as a patient, if you see another sufferer apparently being let down you can begin to lose your faith in the system.

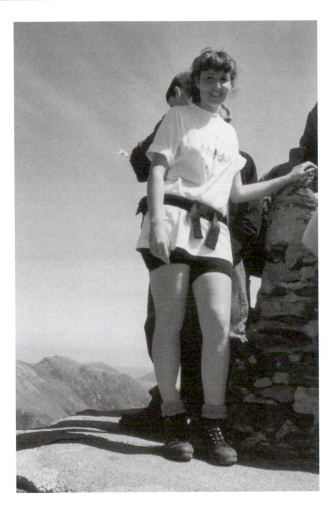

Figure 10   At the top of Snowdon

6   More alternative remedies, such as homeopathic, should be encouraged. There is now a huge market for such things and if something may work then maybe we should try them. Similarly, encouragement to try a new hobby or time to reflect spiritually may also help.

7   A supportive family and friends can never be underestimated. It is very, very hard for the immediate family to cope, particularly with a mentally ill person. The whole family needs to be reminded that they will get better in time and to talk to each other for support. My parents [see Figure 11] continue to be a great help to Nick and I. For the sufferer, it is the apparently

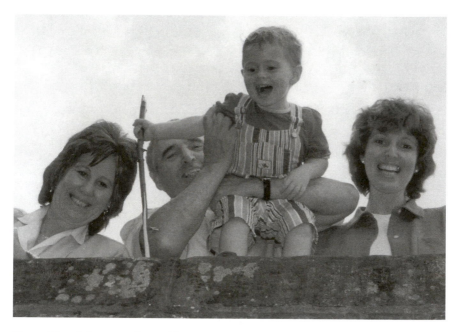

Figure 11   A happy outing with my parents

> small touches that can make a huge impact upon you. One of
> my best friends knew I would not answer the phone but she
> would regularly just ring and chat away on the answerphone,
> hoping that I would be listening. I often was and it was a big
> step one day when I actually picked it up to talk back.
> Another friend used to send me little 'thought' cards which
> also were a tonic. I still read them today.

One enormous area that I am surprised has not been identified as a
key benchmarking area is that of communication. Often
complaints about procedures are due to lack of information leading
to possible misunderstandings. As patients we need to be told about
our care, treatment and medication. Even if you know, we often do
not.

This is especially applicable to first-time mums who can be very
naïve [see Figure 12]. As midwives, you obviously deal with
matters of birth and childcare every day, but to those of us who
are new to it the obvious does need stating. Bear in mind that it is
better to be told something four times than not at all.

I also feel that staff, patients and visitors would benefit in
general by a hospital prospectus at each bed, like in hotels, to
explain who is who, routines, etc.

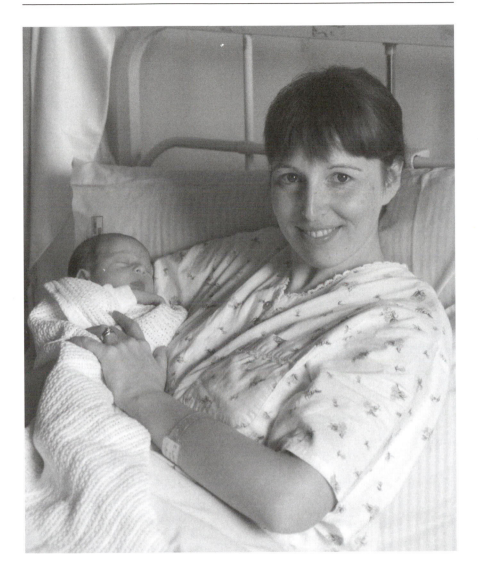

Figure 12 A mum at last

Good communication skills help make a good nurse. It is really appreciated if a nurse shows interest in your cards and flowers, asks about your family and generally treats you as an interesting person. The nurses I remember the most were those who told me a little about themselves.

As patients and families we need to be kept informed of progress and treatments, but this must be realistic. I felt very uneasy when a nurse told me that my grandfather would be moving to a hospice and he would be allowed home for tea occasionally. At that stage he was suffering badly as an 89-year-old dying of lung cancer and I just wanted his pain to end. Giving us false hope was not helpful but being reassured that he would be made as comfortable as possible was.

I am aware of the importance of case conferences for the treatment of some patients; however, please bear in mind that they can be a horrendous ordeal for some patients and families. At my worst in the psychiatric hospital I went in to see the doctor and was faced with about eight professionals – very scary when talking to one person was such an ordeal.

I would like to conclude with a few general points about nursing which have mattered to me as a patient and as a relative:

- When Dominic was so poorly as a baby [see Figure 13] I appreciated being able to stay with him in hospital. Not only did it give me support but hopefully I was able to help in his care and treatment. As parents, please continue to involve us for the mutual benefit of everyone concerned.
- Although a new, purpose-built hospital environment is

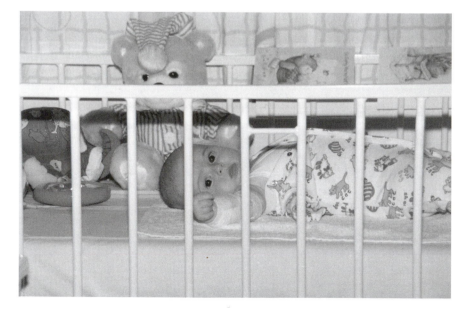

Figure 13   A poorly baby

supposed to be idyllic, the most memorable features for a patient are actually the care and attention given by staff. The ward I spent two months in was an old Victorian asylum, but it was clean, practical and comfortable. At the time it felt like a haven from the rest of the world that I could not cope with. People, not places, are ultimately important.

- The environment can be improved, however, with flowers and personal touches, but as a nurse you can make a difference to patients having to suffer the annoying racket of a television all day long. Turn them down or off!

- Wards obviously need cleaning but do the rotas have to be so early? Often I was disturbed by the thwack of a brush on my bed or the clatter of the bin being emptied. Sleep is supposed to be a good healer, so why in hospitals do there seem to be schemes to stop patients from doing it?

- If we do something wrong in hospital, such as carrying our newborn baby instead of wheeling him in the crib, please reprimand us gently. A short, sharp passing comment from a nurse can deeply upset you when you feel so vulnerable.

- Why do so many health workers smoke? It seems so farcical that every hospital entrance is littered with staff and patients having a quick fix when the wards are full of people suffering the effects of it.

- What really matter to patients are the simplest of actions. Even if you are run off your feet, a passing smile is a real lift. Be gentle with us, mentally and physically, but make us smile or laugh. Compliments are always welcome, especially during observations. Sympathise but be optimistic. A squeeze or pat of the hand and straightening of the bedclothes can be just as valuable as a drug. Inform, reassure, prepare and if you make us feel special, I guarantee we will think you are.

- Remember how you felt as a sick child – poorly but warm, clean and comfortable; your favourite things around you, safe and loved. I was lucky as that was how my mother made me feel and she would have made an excellent nurse.

- One huge factor is to be able to spend time with patients. I can hear the cries of 'If only!' Maybe that is where you can come in Minister. Patients want more good nurses and one way to improve this is to employ more and pay them more. Better pay and conditions would improve the calibre of staff and thus healing rates.

So I hope I have mentioned some areas today which you can act upon. I have possibly picked upon more negative aspects then

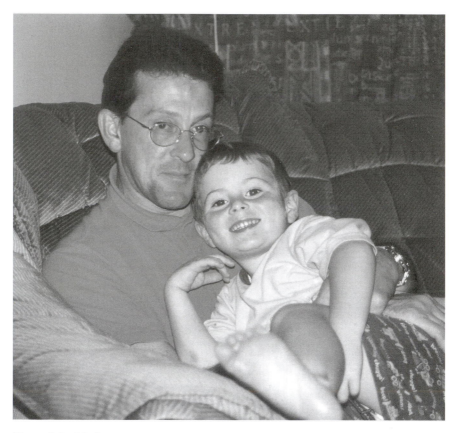

Figure 14 My boys

positive to motivate you all into wanting to make a difference. The National Health Service has enabled me to make such a good recovery and for that I am eternally grateful.

This husband and son [see Figure 14] I am told would have been left without me in years gone by, as I would have been put away in an institution and never been allowed out again. Instead, thanks to the wonderful nursing support and services, we now have a life together which is definitely worth living.

Nursing has made a difference to us. Please carry on and let it do the same for others.

Thank you.'

I was greeted by rapturous applause and noticed many people wiping their eyes again. I had done it! I had just informed nurses from the length and breadth of the country all about my illness. Maybe if it stopped just one from making a sharp remark to a patient then it had been worth it. I was congratulated by many including the conference Chairwoman who praised me both publicly and privately. Mandie looked delighted through her tears and squeezed my arm as I sat back down beside her. 'I knew you could do it,' she said.

After a couple more speakers there was a coffee break. I could not get to the toilets for being stopped and thanked by people. It seemed weird that all these people knew who I was but I did not know them. One lady approached me and said she was a nursing lecturer. She said she felt every student nurse should hear my messages and if I were to write a book it should go on their compulsory reading list. Others too said that they wanted their colleagues to listen to me, and yes, they wanted to know more. Since I had begun talking to people in general about my illness, I found it surprising how many people would then own up to their own mental health problem or someone close to them. It is very much a closed subject until someone dares to break it open. Apparently that is what I had succeeded in doing and for that my courage was recognised and praised. I did not do it for that reason but was glad if it was helpful. I sat in the ladies feeling very tired but very happy. I think I was too drained at this point to feel the elation I had anticipated. That came later on.

Back in the auditorium speakers continued, behind schedule due to the train problems. Hence lunch was going to be later than planned. Mandie kept her eye on the time and before the official break we sneaked out, collected my bags and hailed a taxi for me. She thanked me profusely and wished me a brilliant afternoon as I deserved it. The traffic was bad again due to the problem on the underground but the driver did a valiant job of traversing side streets to get me to the television studio. I made it in time to join a very strange group of people queuing outside. There were all shapes, sizes, nationalities and ages. Some had tickets booked weeks ago, others like me had come for Lionel. I excitedly phoned my mother to tell her I was in the queue. She enquired about a speech – what speech? A young lady with a clipboard asked our names and checked us off against her list. A few minutes later she came back with postcards upon which we had to write a question for Lionel. Mandie and I had come up with one: 'You have written so many beautiful love songs about adults; now you have young children of your own, can you write one that expresses parental love?' I duly wrote it down with my name and handed it back. A few minutes later the young lady returned and my name was the second of five which she read out.

The chosen five were then directed into the studio and strategically positioned. As number two I was on the front row on the right-hand side. The rest of the audience of about 50 wandered in and took their places. I had put my cases and coat to the side and had reapplied my lipstick! The floor manager gave us some house rules and we had to practice clapping and cheering. The show was going out live and within minutes the presenter had welcomed us and final preparations were made. Lionel appeared towards the back of the set and I heard someone shout his name as they waved. Oops, it was me. He looked up and waved back! The confident woman who had just delivered an emotional speech to hundreds of nurses was now a drooling pop fanatic! The show went out live and I was in an absolute shock and delirium as my all-time music star was sitting at a grand piano, no more than five feet away from me, singing a ballad from his new album. Several times he caught my fixed stare on him and smiled directly at me as he sang.

A few other guests were interviewed and there were a couple of commercial breaks, during which the floor staff ran around changing sets, etc. During one of them Lionel stood next to the floor manager who had a list on his clipboard of the people who were going to ask him the questions. As they read each one the particular audience member was pointed out and Lionel glanced up at them. I was still broadly grinning as he looked me straight in the eye for 'number 2'. He smiled at me again. During his actual interview, live on air, if he glanced towards the autocue all he could see was my head above it still with a stupid grin on it! I was so glad no one there knew me. Maybe my infantile behaviour was a reaction to the stress of the morning – maybe not. The show progressed and for the umpteenth time I checked my hair, read the question on the card I was sitting on and waited for 'number 2' to be spoken to. They also had phone calls and questions from viewers which he answered. Then it was 'number 1's' turn. My heart pounded as I knew I would be next, and I rehearsed yet again my question. The presenter, Gloria Hunniford, then announced, 'That's all we've got time for. Thank you ...'

What? Was that it? What about the rest of our questions? With that the show ended, the credits rolled and the floor manager began to usher people out. A few people had surrounded Lionel and he was signing autographs. I stayed in my seat, stunned and *so* disappointed. The floor manager passed by me and I could not help myself from indignantly saying to him, 'Well! That wasn't very nice! You have worked five of us up to ask Lionel a question and did not tell us at any time that you might not be able to include us all. And now we're just expected to go?'

He looked amazed and mildly apologised something about time running out. Meanwhile everyone was being encouraged to go. Not me. I stood up, smoothed my dress down and walked straight through the small crowd of fans around Lionel. I stood in front of him, placed my hand on his chest and said, 'You're my hero. Your music has been with me through good and bad times, through college days and a divorce. I'm now happily married again and have a son. Please will you write a song about children? It would be wonderful in your hands!'

He looked me straight in the eye, smiled, stroked my cheek with his finger and kissed me, saying, 'That's a beautiful idea and I'll do my best.'

I floated back to my coat and bags, saying to myself, 'Lionel Richie just kissed me!' I wanted to hug the floor manager but he just looked at me gingerly and headed off in another direction. Once I got outside into the cold, crisp air, I fastened my jacket up and looked at the time. I still had at least an hour before my train was due and I knew the station was only a few minutes way. A large, black car was parked at the main studio door. I asked the driver if he was waiting for Lionel and he admitted he was. So I just had to wait, didn't I? In the interim, members of the band came and went in another car and a small gathering of other fans hovered around the doorway. I stayed by the original car. In yet another moment of madness I scribbled on the back of one of our name and address cards that my little boy was called Dominic, and a reminder to write a song about children. I asked the chauffeur if he could give it to Lionel and he placed it on the back seat.

At last we all could see Lionel and his entourage through the glass walls and he came out, dressed head to toe in black and wearing dark glasses. He signed some autographs, posed for some photographs and smiled at me as

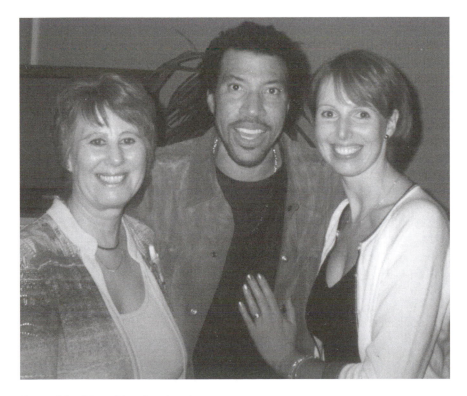

Figure 15 Mum, Lionel and me!

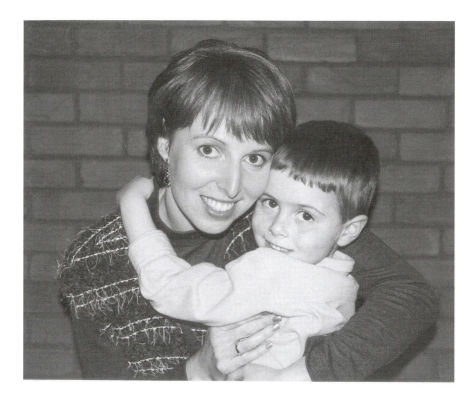

Figure 16   Sparkly eyes at last

he got into his car. It began to move away, then I saw Lionel reach forward to the driver and the car stopped. The darkened glass window slowly came down and Lionel looked back towards me and shouted my name. He said he had got my note; that he would write a song about children and it would be just for me! With that he kissed my hand and the car disappeared into the London rush-hour traffic, leaving me even more stunned. I now had a cheek and hand that had been kissed by him. What a charmer. Even if he was humouring me, I cannot wait for his next album to come out! A few months later my mother and I met him again, backstage after a concert [see Figure 15].

In a daze I found my way back to the station and managed to get Dominic a Union Jack t-shirt for his current patriotic phase. I went into the first-class lounge and had a drink and some biscuits. I realised then that I had not eaten since breakfast. The journey home was efficient and my fellow passenger, a sales representative from the Midlands, made the mistake of asking me what I had been doing in London. Did I have a tale to tell him. As he disembarked he said he looked forward to my book. When people at home enquired about my speech they hardly heard about it – just the Lionel part. My head teacher made the comment that she had not given me leave to cavort with pop stars – she was smiling though!

I had been to London; I had spoken to all those nurses. I was better and now both my son and I definitely have sparkly eyes [see Figure 16]! Now I shall get on with my life with Nick and Dominic and all those people who make the world a better place by just being in it.

CHAPTER 26

Insight into emotional disorders associated with childbirth

Thelma Osborn

Emotional disorders

Pregnancy and childbirth are universally perceived to be happy events. However, for some women this is not the case. Some women may experience emotional, psychological and physical difficulties in the postnatal period. The result is sadness, unhappiness and pain affecting the woman and her significant others including her child/ren.

There are three childbirth-related emotional disorders: the blues, postnatal depression and puerperal psychosis (PP).

The blues

The blues affect around 50–70% of all women,[1,2] occurring usually within the first ten days of delivery. The trigger for the blues is thought to be hormonal.[3] Research has shown that a sudden drop in hormonal levels following delivery sets off an emotional response. Some women are more sensitive to these hormonal changes and may exhibit varying degrees of responses. Women can become quite tearful, irritable, easily upset and distressed and anxious around the baby.

Treatment

There is no need for medication. This short emotional episode responds well to rest, support and reassurance by family and/or professionals. However, approximately 50% of women who are severely affected by the blues will go on to become depressed. So, close surveillance by family and health professionals, with follow-up, is important.

Postnatal depression

Postnatal depression affects around 10–15% of women in the first postnatal year and beyond.[4,5] It is usually recognised in the first six months of the postnatal period.

Symptoms

Symptoms include:

- low mood and sadness
- tearfulness
- feelings of worthlessness
- self-blame or guilt
- anxiety
- irritability with emotional highs and lows
- lack of energy, lack of interest in activities
- feelings of hopelessness
- confused thoughts
- sleep-disturbances (unrelated to the baby)
- changes in appetite
- reduced concentration and difficulty making decisions
- worries about their own and the baby's health
- loss of interest in sex
- thoughts about death and suicide. Very rarely women have contemplated or attempted suicide and/or had obsessional thoughts about harming the baby.

The unhappy, irritable, tired, tearful mother is easily recognisable, but there are others whose symptoms are less recognisable. Symptoms may not always be expressed. Some women can be quite good at masking their difficulties: 'the smiling depressive'. These women may seek help with physical complaints such as headache, backache and pain in various areas, or difficulties with the baby such as crying/settling, feeding and sleeping.

Postnatal depression is classified as mild, moderate or severe. The level of depression will determine the most appropriate type of intervention. Most important is early identification followed by appropriate management.

It is important to be aware that women can become depressed and anxious in the antenatal period, with similar symptoms to those of postnatal depression. Regardless of the level and time of onset of depression, it can be very distressing and disabling to the mother, and her family and friends. It can also have a negative effect on marital relationships, the mother–infant relationship, child behaviour and the child's intellectual development.[6–9]

So, how do we treat and detect anxiety and depression related to childbirth? It is helpful to be aware of the possible causes as it helps identify potential women and inform suitable intervention.

Causes

Many studies have been undertaken to determine the possible causes and risk factors of postnatal depression. Those identified are often referred to under the headings of biological, social and psychological causes.

However, in my experience women relate better to specific named causes, such as:

- disturbed early life
- loss of own mother
- current marital or family conflicts
- infertility and investigations for four years or more
- loss of a previous pregnancy or baby from stillbirth or cot death
- adoption or fostering
- high medical anxieties over the pregnancy
- admission to hospital for longer than one week in the last three months of pregnancy
- major upheavals or stresses in the last three months of pregnancy such as moving house
- emergency Caesarean section
- neonatal illnesses – especially separation and admission of baby to neonatal unit
- major upheaval and stresses in the first three months after delivery
- hormonal changes
- personal or family history of depression.

A list of this nature can perhaps seem quite frightening to the outsider. However women are often relieved to know that there are reasons why they are feeling, thinking, or behaving in a particular way.

Detection

Health visitors or general practitioners (GPs) are uniquely placed to identify women with postnatal depression/emotional disorders. Both professionals for various reasons, see mothers routinely in the first postnatal year. If suitably trained and skilled, these professionals are able to work as a team in detecting and managing this condition within the community/primary care setting.

Professionals such as health visitors, midwives, and general practitioners need to be trained in accurate mood assessment, to be aware of the signs and symptoms of postnatal depression and how women may present themselves. They would then be able to make early identification and so shorten the distress caused by this condition.

To assist in detection, various screening tools have been developed. These tools, such as the Edinburgh Postnatal Depression Scale,[10] may be used by trained professionals in conjunction with clinical assessment to assist in identifying women with postnatal depression. It is also important that an accurate history is taken, as this forms part of the clinical assessment. As stated earlier there are times when detection is simple as symptoms are easily recognisable. But some women will mask symptoms for reasons such as fear of being stigmatised, ashamed of people's reactions, being labelled as not coping or mad, or having their children/baby taken away.

There is still a stigma attached to depression. Recently the stigma has lessened because of celebrities and royals, such as the late Princess of Wales, being identified as suffering from postnatal depression. Women therefore feel less shameful about their negative reactions to childbirth and there is more openness within the general public.

Management

Three aspects of care/treatment that have proven to be helpful are listening, social support and antidepressants. Listening is by way of one-to-one counselling, ideally by a specialist counsellor/trained professional or health visitor, trained in 'listening visits and cognitive behaviour therapy'.[11] Some women find postnatal depression therapy groups helpful. Family support and social support is also highly beneficial. There are voluntary or statutory organisations providing support, such as Sure Start, mother and toddler groups, National Childbirth Trust – these have all proved to be a great source of help for many women.

Antidepressants, prescribed by their GP, may also be required for some women. However, women need to be made aware that antidepressants can take up to two weeks to work and are generally non-addictive. Antidepressants should be taken until recovery and then for at least six months afterwards to prevent relapse. On the very rare occasions when there is a significant likelihood of harm or actual harm to the baby, social services may become involved for a short period to provide extra help and support.

Puerperal psychosis

Puerperal psychosis (PP) is the most severe and worrying disturbance following childbirth. It is rare, affecting 1–2 women per thousand, and normally onsets within the first four postnatal weeks.[12,13] Women may suddenly develop an anxious and variable mood, with mania or depression. They may experience difficulty sleeping, disordered thinking, paranoia, agitation, confusion, and have ideas of harming themselves or the baby, which are sometimes acted out. There may be serious risk of suicide or infanticide.

The law recognises that some women become severely emotionally disturbed after the birth of a child. The Infanticide Act of 1938 states that a woman cannot be found guilty of manslaughter if she kills her own child within twelve months of birth provided 'the balance of her mind was disturbed by reason of her not having fully recovered from the effects of giving birth'.

PP occurs more often in younger, first-time mothers with a past personal or family history of psychosis, whose babies were delivered by Caesarean section. It is also likely to be hormone related. A previous history of PP increases the likelihood of recurrence by 50%. Women with bipolar disorder are also at high risk of recurrence following delivery.

Treatment

PP is normally best treated in hospital, in a specialised mother and baby unit where expert care is provided. In hospital, women may fail to recognise family members and may not realise that they are in hospital. There may be psychotic symptoms such as delusions and hallucinations, bewilderment and disorientation in time, place and person.

After careful mental health assessment, and if there are good community support services, care in the community may be possible. In the community the mother will require a great deal of supervision and encouragement from mental health teams, primary care teams and from family and friends.

If treated in hospital, a special mother and baby unit helps to decrease the mother's level of anxiety, keeps her in touch with reality and preserves the bonding between mother and baby. However, there are few specialist units in the country. Women respond well to treatment with antipsychotics and antidepressants. Occasionally, electroconvulsive therapy (ECT) is appropriate. A full recovery is usual.

Like postnatal depression, PP can also have a negative effect on relationships with significant others and the mother–infant relationship. It is a most distressing time for the woman, her family and friends.

On the very rare occasions when there is significant likelihood of harm or actual harm to the baby, social services may become involved for a short period to provide extra help and support.

Personal interest

I qualified as a Registered General Nurse, Midwife and Health Visitor in the mid- and late-seventies. In the mid-nineties I qualified with an MA in counselling, with postnatal depression as my research subject. For the last 14 years I have worked in the field of postnatal mental health.

Student nurses in general training are taught little about mental health or midwifery as part of the general curriculum. These are viewed as specialist areas. Students in general nursing are given the opportunity to gain insight into such specialist fields by way of a few weeks of attachment experience. As a second year student, I worked for three months secondment in a psychiatric hospital and three months in a maternity unit of a general hospital. This was unusual as one was usually offered only one of these secondments. My taster sessions in these two units caused a dilemma in my choice of specialty. In the end, the maternity unit was a catalyst for my midwifery training.

My midwifery training was exceptional as there were few trainees in a very busy unit. We learnt quickly – there were even staff shortages in those days! I became theoretically aware of all the physical and emotional effects of pregnancy and childbirth, including assessment procedures, interventions and management of normal and abnormal pregnancy, labour, delivery and postnatal care. Learning is about gaining knowledge. Skills develop from an ability to put knowledge into action and to be effective. Looking back as a newly-qualified midwife, my skills relating to the physical care of my patients/clients and their families were excellent. It was some time before I developed the skills to become emotionally/mentally in tune with clients.

Generally, antenatal and postnatal women then and now have sparkling eyes. If for some reason there are difficulties that interfere with this sparkle, most women appear to have an innate ability to create an artificial sparkle. A mask. The result is that their emotional needs are unmet, or there can be a considerable delay in getting these needs met. An artificial sparkle or mask can be so very effective that a professional, or a confiding family or friend may be unsuccessful in getting behind that mask.

My first experience of supporting a woman with PP was while working as a staff midwife in a busy postnatal ward some 20 years ago. What stood out for me was the sudden and intense onset of symptoms. They were typical of PP – anxious and variable mood with mania and depression, difficulty in sleeping, disordered thinking, paranoia, agitation, confusion, ideas of self-harm and harming the baby, failure to recognise family members, bewilderment and disorientation in time, place and person. This was a most distressing time for the woman and her family and for the staff. It is a part of midwifery that no textbook can adequately prepare a midwife for. The whole family needed support. This woman was treated as an in-patient and made a full recovery. I sometimes think about this family; the baby is now perhaps a parent.

Contact with the author/my impressions

The author contacted me by telephone and asked if I would be willing to read and then write a foreword to a book she was writing about her mental health experiences following the birth of her child. I agreed and she duly posted the manuscript to me. The title was *Eyes Without Sparkle*.

From start to finish my impression was that it was a brilliant script and a book which would be helpful for professionals and non-professionals. Another impression was that it was about someone who had experienced the most rare and difficult form of postnatal illnesses – puerperal psychosis – and was telling her story in a real and moving way. I admired her courage tremendously.

I met with the author for the first time a few weeks after reading her script. I apologised for saying that I enjoyed reading about her experiences – she understood what I meant. I congratulated her on her openness and the way she brought the entire script of her life at that time 'into life'. Later on, I was delighted when she asked me to write this chapter.

From the start the script was easy reading, enjoyable, informative and friendly. However, the author seemed to be constantly busy in her daily life. I wanted to say to her, 'Stop! Have a break, you are doing too much'. I felt that she would not be able to maintain such an active lifestyle, that she was heading for a collapse of some kind. I would like to have got behind the mask of her businesses, to explore her thoughts, feelings, and behaviour with her. I would also have liked to explore with her the possibility of rest, taking time out for herself and doing some pleasant and pleasurable things.

It was some considerable time before there was complete failure of her coping mechanisms. She was admitted to hospital, eight months postnatal in a collapsed, agitated and exhausted state.

It took sometime before the mask disappeared and her eyes completely ceased to sparkle.

Sometimes for us professionals it's about developing the skills for getting behind that mask and recognising the sadness under the smiles, and questioning and exploring with the mother her busy lifestyle or apparent lack of social life, isolation, sadness and, for some, the traumatic effects and experiences of pregnancy, labour and delivery. It can be extremely helpful for mothers to have the opportunity to talk to a trained professional about her thoughts and feelings, including loss that motherhood can evoke – her anger, fears, anxieties, beliefs, hopes and expectations.

A trained professional with a high degree of sensitivity, who is able to contain and understand the turmoil that some women experience and offer appropriate supportive interventions, enables the establishment of a satisfactory and helping relationship. This relationship allows a woman to be open and honest about her difficulties. The result is the development of a working partnership with women to enable them to develop or redevelop the ability to enjoy life and parenting and ensure that their eyes remain sparkling.

Postnatal mental illness has a story. Some stories are simple and others quite complex. Help, support and interventions need to match the story line. That's why it is important to have an accurate assessment so that women are given the right kind of help and support at the earliest possible time.

The author appears to have some positive and negative experiences of the services she received. Hospital seemed to be particularly unpleasant for her. In hospital her treatment was by major tranquillisers, antidepressants and ECT. Family and friends were a vital part of the healing process. She would have been under the care of a consultant psychiatrist in a psychiatric unit. There were bonding issues. Separation from the baby while in hospital, as he was cared for at home, might have increased these problems. In addition, the separation would not have helped her anxious state or disorientation. We know that nationally there are limited specialist mother and baby units for maternal mental health problems.

On very rare occasions when there is actual harm to a baby or likelihood of harm, social services may get involved. The aim of their involvement is to ensure the safety of the baby, and to offer much help and support to the woman and her family, and to maintain a family unit. Social services will work closely with all other professionals, parents and significant others. Parents will be invited to meetings and will be part of the decision-making process. The author appears to have coped quite well with social services involvement, including home visits, meetings and action plans.

Due to the nature of her illness, when she was discharged from hospital, in addition to the health visitor's continual support, she was also under the care of the community mental health services. The community mental health nurse would maintain regular contact through home visits and outpatient consultations. The psychiatrist at outpatient clinics would also have seen her on regular occasions.

A care plan would have been agreed before her discharge from hospital. There is a likelihood that there would have been professionals meeting before discharge, with the community mental health team, primary care teams and other relevant professionals involved in her care invited. She and her personal support network – significant family or friends – would also be a part of these interchanges. From the onset, her GP would be kept informed of her care and mental health involvement, as eventually she would be discharged completely into the care of her GP.

In the event of more than one professional or agency being involved in the care of a woman, it is important that the lines of communication are open and clear to everyone. It is essential that the woman and her family are part of the decision-making process. A key worker would be assigned to ensure there is a named person for the woman and her family to contact with any concerns. Also, another responsibility of this key worker would be monitoring the woman's wellbeing, and ensuring that any planned help/ support/intervention is completed.

Three main emotional difficulties have been highlighted in this chapter. The Government has recently sought, through various legislation, to improve the health and social functioning of women and their families in the early years through a number of services. Antenatal and postnatal mental healthcare has been highlighted as needing to be rapid, appropriate, accessible and effective, being provided by health professionals possessing appropriate skills, experiences and resources.

Nine out of ten mothers will have a satisfactory postnatal period. For those who experience a depressive episode, whose eyes are not sparkling, it can be a traumatic time for all concerned, with negative implications, especially for the mother, her child and partner.

It is important that in the antenatal and postnatal periods there is adequate and appropriate emotional and social support. Professionals need to be trained to identify vulnerable women early. I hope this book will inform trainee and trained professionals and non-professionals about postnatal mental disorders. Provision for care, whether it is emotional, physical, social, or medication, should be of a high and appropriate standard. The negative mental health effects of childbirth need to be prevented or reduced, and mothers' eyes will be forever sparkling.

References

1 Kendell RE, McGuire RJ, Connor Y *et al.* (1981) Mood changes in the first three weeks after childbirth. *Journal of Affective Disorders.* **3**: 317–26.

2 Stein G, Marsh A and Morton J (1981) Mental symptoms, weight changes and electrolyte excretion during the first postpartum week. *Journal of Psychosomatic Research.* **25**: 395–408.

3 Nott PN, Franklin M, Armitage C *et al.* (1976) Hormonal changes and mood in puerperium. *British Journal of Psychiatry.* **128**: 379–83.

4 Cox J, Connor Y and Kendall R (1982) Prospective study of the psychiatry disorders of childbirth. *British Journal of Psychiatry.* **140**: 782–6.

5 Kumar R and Robson K (1984) A prospective study of the emotional disorders in childbearing women. *British Journal of Psychiatry.* **144**: 35–47.

6 Sharpe D, Hale D, Pawlby S *et al.* (1995) The impact of postnatal depression on boys' intellectual development. *Journal of Child Psychology and Psychiatry.* **36**: 8.

7 Murray L (1992) The impact of postnatal depression on infant development. *Journal of Psychology and Psychiatry.* **33**: 543–61.

8 Caplan J, Cogill S, Alexandra H *et al.* (1989) Maternal depression and the emotional development of the child. *British Journal of Psychiatry.* **154**: 818–23.

9 Cogill S, Caplan H, Alexandra H *et al.* (1986) Impact of postnatal depression on cognitive development of young children. *British Medical Journal.* **292**: 1165–7.

10 Cox JL, Holden J and Sagovsky R (1987) Detection of postnatal depression; development of the 10-item Edinburgh postnatal scale. *British Journal of Psychiatry.* **150**: 782–6.

11 Holden J, Sagovsky R and Cox J (1989) Counselling in a general practice setting: controlled study of health visitors' intervention in treatment of postnatal depression. *British Journal of Psychiatry.* **298**: 223–6.

12 Kendall R, Chalmers JC and Platz C (1987) Epidemiology of puerperal psychosis. *British Journal of Psychiatry.* **150**: 662–73.

13 Paffenbarger R (1964) Epidemiological aspects of postpartum mental illness. *British Journal of Preventive Social Medicine.* **18**: 189–95.

Appendix

Books and publications

Aiken C (2000) *Surviving Post Natal Depression.* Jessica Kingsley, London.

Barnett B (1990) *Coping with Postnatal Depression.* Penguin, Sydney.

Bennett S and Indman P (2003) *Beyond the Blues: a guide to understanding and treating prenatal and postpartum depression.* Moodswings Press, San Jose, CA.

Bishop L (1999) *Postnatal Depression: families in turmoil.* Halstead Press, Rushcutters Bay.

Brockington I (1996) *Motherhood and Mental Health.* Oxford University Press, New York.*

Cohen D (2002) *The Father's Book: being a good dad in the 21st century.* John Wiley & Sons Inc., New York.

Comport M (1997) *Towards Happy Motherhood: understanding postnatal depression.* Corgi/The Guernsey Press Co., Guernsey, Channel Isles.

Cox J and Holden J (2003) *Perinatal Mental Health: a guide to the Edinburgh Postnatal Depression Scale.* Gaskell (Royal College of Psychiatrists), London.

Curham S (2000) *Antenatal and Postnatal Depression: practical advice and support for all sufferers.* Vermilion, London.

Dalton K and Holton W (1999) *Once a Month: understanding and treating PMS.* Hunter House, Inc., xxx, CA.

Dalton K and Holton W (ed) (2001) *Depression After Childbirth: how to recognise, treat and prevent postnatal depression.* Oxford University Press, New York.

Dix C (1985) *The New Mother Syndrome: coping with postpartum stress and depression.* Pocket Books, New York.

Dix C (1987) *The New Mother Syndrome: coping with postnatal stress and depression.* Allen & Unwin, St Leonards, NSW.

Dunnewold A and Sanford DG (1994) *Postpartum Survival Guide.* New Harbinger Publications, Oakland, CA.

Fettling L (2002) *Postnatal Depression: a practical guide for Australian families.* IP Communications, East Hawthorn, Melbourne.

Huysman AM (2003) *The Postpartum Effect: deadly depression in mothers.* Seven Stories Press, New York.

Kendall-Tackett KA (2001) *The Hidden Feelings of Motherhood: a guide to coping with stress, depression, and burnout.* New Harbinger Publications, Oakland, CA.

Kitzinger S (1994) *The Year After Childbirth: surviving and enjoying the first year of motherhood.* Charles Scribner's Sons, New York.

Kleinman K and Raskin VD (1994) *This Isn't What I Expected: recognizing and recovering from depression and anxiety after childbirth.* Bantam, Doubleday Dell Pub Inc, New York.

Marshall F (1993) *Coping with post-natal depression.* Sheldon Press, London.

Milgrom J, Martin PR and Negri LM (2000) *Treating Postnatal Depression: a psychological approach for healthcare practitioners.* John Wiley and Sons Ltd, Chichester and New York.

MIND (2003) *Understanding Post-natal Depression.* MIND, London.

Misri S (1995) *Shouldn't I Be Happy.* Free Press – Simon and Schuster, New York.

Nicolson P (2001) *Postnatal depression: facing the paradox of loss, happiness and motherhood.* John Wiley and Sons Ltd, Chichester and New York.

Osmond M (2001) *Behind the Smile: my journey out of postpartum depression.* Warner Books, New York.

Pacific Post Partum Support Society (1987) *Post Partum Depression and Anxiety.* Pacific Post Partum Support Society, Vancouver.

Polden M and Whiteford B (1992) *The Postnatal Exercise Book.* Frances Lincoln, London.

Riley D (1995) *Perinatal Mental Health: a source book for health professionals.* Radcliffe Medical Press, Oxford.

Sapsted A (1990) *Banish Post Baby Blues.* Thorsons Publishing, Wellingborough.

Scott D (2001) *Making Mummy Better: a child's experience of postnatal depression.* Spectrum Publications, Melbourne.

Stern D *et al.* (1999) *The Birth of a Mother: how motherhood changes you forever.* Basic Books, New York, Canada and Australia.

Weekes C (1995) *Self-Help for your Nerves.* HarperCollins, London.

Welburn V (1980) *Postnatal Depression.* Manchester University Press, Manchester.

Welford H (2002) *The NCT Book of Postnatal Depression: feelings after birth.* NCT Publishing, Cambridge.*

Wolf N (2003) *Misconceptions: truth, lies and the unexpected on the journey to motherhood.* Anchor Books, New York.

Visit www.ppdsupportpage.com/book.html for a useful link to many US books.

---

*Contains further reading on Puerperal Psychosis. The Association for Post Natal Illness and Meet-A-Mum Association (*see* pp 228 and 234) both publish leaflets about puerperal psychosis.

There is a video available called *Understanding Post Natal Depression* by Liz Wise, an experienced PND counsellor. It can be ordered by writing to: PND Productions, 13 Barnett Row, Jacobswell, Guildford GU4 7PH, UK or by e-mailing: lwise@onetel.net.uk or by visiting: www.postnataldepression.com. Tel: +44(0)7745 113197.

Organisations and agencies for further information and support

Although I have found these references I have not evaluated them and I do not accept responsibility for the information nor the quality of the information contained on these sites.

4women
Website: www.crosswire.karoo.net/4women.htm
A website designed by sufferers of postnatal depression who want to raise awareness and dispel the myths that surround PND, as well as to help other sufferers and offer information. Includes a well-used and trusted forum. Access via address above or through a link from www.motherwise. co.uk.

Action on Puerperal Psychosis
Website: www.neuroscience.bham.ac.uk/research/app/
The University of Birmingham has established Action on Puerperal Psychosis (APP), a network of women who have suffered puerperal psychosis and who are willing to receive correspondence from them about research projects. As puerperal psychosis is a relatively uncommon disorder (affecting about one in 1000 deliveries), it can be difficult to find enough sufferers to carry out effective research and APP is an important resource for researchers. There are plans to transfer this unit to the University of Wales.

Association for Improvements in the Maternity Services (AIMS)
5 Ann's Court, Grove Road, Surbiton, Surrey KT6 4BE, UK
Tel: +44 (0)870 765 1453; fax: +44 (0)870 765 1454
Website: www.aims.org.uk; e-mail: Chair@aims.org.uk
Pressure group founded in 1966. Membership is mainly parents, but includes many in midwifery and medical professions. Offers information, support and advice about all aspects of maternity care, including parents' rights, choices and so on. Also available: information leaflets and a quarterly journal.

Association for Post Natal Illness
145 Dawes Road, Fulham, London SW6 7EB, UK

Helpline: +44 (0)20 7386 0868
Website: www.apni.org; e-mail: info@apni.org
This organisation provides support to mothers suffering from postnatal illness. It exists to increase public awareness of the illness and to encourage research into its cause and nature. It also offers a range of leaflets and its website has some excellent links to other PND websites.

Association of Breastfeeding Mothers
PO Box 207, Bridgwater, Somerset TA6 7YT, UK
Helpline: +44 0870 401 7711
Website: www.abm.me.uk/; e-mail: info@abm.me.uk
Support and information about breastfeeding.

AWARE
72 Lower Leeson Street, Dublin 2, Republic of Ireland
Tel: +353 (0)1 661 7211; fax: +353 (0)1 661 7217; lo-call helpline: 1890 303 302
Website: www.aware.ie; e-mail: info@aware.ie
AWARE is a voluntary organisation, based in Ireland, formed in 1985 by a group of interested patients, relatives and mental health professionals, whose aims are to assist that section of the population whose lives are directly affected by depression. There is a useful section specifically on post-natal depression.

BabyCentre
Website: www.babycentre.co.uk; e-mail: uk_feedback@babycentre.co.uk
The UK's hands-on guide to pregnancy, birth and life. A useful site with a great deal of information, support and reassurance on these matters with specific areas about postnatal illness. They have US sister sites of Baby-Center and ParentsCenter.

Baby-Parenting
Website: www.baby-parenting.co.uk
Baby-Parenting.co.uk is a fun website for parents, expectant parents and those trying to conceive. It contains useful information, good links and listings for everything from toy shops to child-care facilities. There are many links on postnatal issues.

Babyworld
Slate Barn, Mongewell Park Farm, Wallingford, Oxon OX10 8BS, UK
Website: www.babyworld.co.uk/; email: contactus@babyworld.co.uk
UK on-line magazine and community, with thousands of pages of help and advice for new and expectant parents. There are links to postnatal issues.

BBC
Website: www.bbc.co.uk/health
There are some helpful pages within this site, including an article asking if fathers can suffer from PND.

Beacon of Hope
Website: www.lightship.org; e-mail: beacon@lightship.org
This site is dedicated to men and women who are partners of someone diagnosed with a severe mental illness. It has very helpful ideas to give everyone support.

Beating the Blues
Ultrasis, 4th Floor, 13–17 Long Lane, London EC1A 9PN, UK
Tel: +44 (0)20 7600 6777.
Website: www.ultrasis.com; e-mail: info@ultrasis.com
A computer-based treatment programme for depression, with clinical supervision.

Beyond the Blues
Shoshana S Bennett PhD, 390 Diablo Road, Suite 115, Danville, CA 94526, USA
Tel: +1 888 484 6667
Websites: www.beyondtheblues.com and www.postpartumassistance.com; e-mail: DrShosh@BeyondTheBlues.com
Both websites give information and support. Full details given about a book entitled *Beyond the Blues*.

BIOME/ MEDLINE/ NMAP
BIOME, University of Nottingham, Greenfield Medical Library, Queens Medical Centre, Nottingham NG7 2UH, UK
Tel: +44 (0)115 849 3251; fax: +44 (0)115 849 3265
Websites: www.biome.ac.uk/; www.omni.ac.uk/medline/; www.nmap.ac.uk/
BIOME offers free access to a searchable catalogue of internet sites and resources covering the health and life sciences. MEDLINE is the US National Library of Medicine's bibliographic database, covering the fields of medicine, nursing, dentistry, veterinary medicine, the healthcare system and the preclinical sciences. It provides access to abstracts of articles and citations from more than 4000 biomedical journals published worldwide. A search for 'postnatal' brings up 32 links to follow. It also links to the NMAP (Nursing, Midwifery and the Allied Health Professions) database, which contains even more links.

Breastfeeding and Childbirth Resources
Website: www.breastfeeding.co.uk; e-mail: jane@breastfeeding.co.uk

Jane's 'Breast-feeding Resources' are a gateway to breast-feeding information, self-help support and books plus other links concerning this and other childbirth and parenting issues.

Breast-feeding Network
The Breast-feeding Network, PO Box 11126, Paisley PA2 8YB, UK
Breast-feeding Network supporter line: +44 (0)870 900 8787
Website: www.breastfeedingnetwork.org.uk; e-mail: email@breastfeeding network.org.uk
An independent source of support and information for breast-feeding women and others.

British Association for Counselling and Psychotherapy (BACP)
BACP House, 35–37 Albert Street, Rugby, Warwickshire CV21 2SG, UK
Tel: +44 (0)870 443 5252; fax: +44 (0)870 443 5161
Websites: www.bacp.co.uk and www.counselling.co.uk; e-mail: bacp@bacp.co.uk
BACP is the professional body for counselling and psychotherapy and an automatic reference point for anyone seeking information on these subjects in the United Kingdom. Send an A5 SAE for details of local practitioners.

Center for Postpartum Health in California
Diana Lynn Barnes Psy.D, MFT, Founder and Director, The Center for Postpartum Health, 20700 Ventura Blvd, Ste. 203, Woodland Hills, CA 91364, USA
Tel: +1 818 887 1312; fax: +1 818 887 9606
Website: www.postpartumhealth.com; e-mail: dlbarnes@postpartumhealth.com
An assessment and treatment centre based in California but it has some links to other resources and information applicable worldwide.

CRY-SIS
27 Old Gloucester Street, London WC1N 3XX, UK
Helpline: +44 (0)20 7404 5011 (7 days a week, 9 a.m.–10 p.m.)
Website: www.cry-sis.com; e-mail: info@cry-sis.org.uk
Cry-sis offers support for families with excessively crying, sleepless and demanding babies. The answering service will give you the phone number of volunteer contacts, who once had similar problems.

Depression Alliance
National Office, 35 Westminster Bridge Road, London SE1 7JB, UK
Tel: +44 (0)20 7633 0557; fax: +44 (0)20 7633 0559; helpline: +44
Information line: 0845 123 2320
Website: www.depressionalliance.org

Depression Alliance is a member-led organisation that co-ordinates a national network of self-help groups and offers a series of free publications, which provide information on depression and related topics. We also offer a range of mutual support services for our members, including a pen friend scheme, correspondence service and email group.

Families online
Website: www.familiesonline.co.uk
An on-line information service for families with young children. There are forums for discussions plus features, reviews, directories, competitions and local information.

Fathers Direct
Herald House, Lambs Passage, Bunhill Row, London, EC1Y 8TQ, UK
Phone: +44 0845 634 1328; fax: +44 (0)20 7374 2966
Website: www.fathersdirect.com; e-mail: webmaster@fathersdirect.com
Fathers Direct is the UK's national information centre for fatherhood. It is a charity founded in 1999 by professionals with expertise in social work, family policy, business development and communications. It exists to support the welfare of children by the positive and active involvement of fathers and male carers in their lives. There is the opportunity here for a forum for fathers on the subject.

Gingerbread
7 Sovereign Close, Sovereign Court, London E1W 2HW, UK
Tel: +44 (0)20 7488 9300; fax: +44 (0)20 7488 9333; advice line and membership freephone: +44 (0)800 018 4318
Website: www.gingerbread.org.uk; e-mail: office@gingerbread.org.uk
This is a support organisation for lone parent families which provides telephone advice and information; a website discussion forum and chat room, and a network of local mutual aid/support groups.

HAPIS
Tel: +44 (0)775 468 7423
Website: www.hapis.org.uk; e-mail: info@hapis.org.uk
An Inverness-based support group for antenatal and postnatal mothers.

Health Education Board for Scotland
NHS Health Scotland, Woodburn House, Canaan Lane, Edinburgh EH10 4SG, UK
Tel: +44 (0)131 536 5500; fax: +44 (0)131 536 5501
Website: www.hebs.scot.nhs.uk; e-mail: publications@hebs.scot.nhs.uk
An informative leaflet about PND.

Home Start
2 Salisbury Road, Leicester LE1 7QR, UK
Tel: +44 (0)116 233 9955; fax: +44 (0)116 233 0232
Free national information line: 0800 068 6368
Website: www.homestart.org.uk; e-mail: info@home-start.org.uk
Home Start volunteers provide free, confidential emotional and practical support and friendship to families in their own homes due to a number of reasons, including postnatal illness, isolation, disability, relationship difficulties and bereavement.

International Society for Psychosomatic Obstetrics and Gynaecology (ISPOG)
Website: www.ispog.org; e-mail: info@ispog.org
ISPOG is an international organisation which aims to promote the study of psychobiological and psychosocial, ethical and cross-cultural problems in the fields of obstetrics and gynaecology, women's health and reproductive health and to encourage the creation of national societies of psychosomatic obstetrics and gynaecology which will promote research, education and training on a national level.

Lactation Consultants of Great Britain
PO Box 56, Virginia Water, Surrey GU25 4WB, UK
Website: www.lcgb.org; e-mail: info@lcgb.org
Facilitating breast-feeding through education, parental support and public health measures.

La Leche League
La Leche League GB, PO Box 29, West Bridgford, Nottingham NG2 7NP, UK
For breast-feeding information and support, call the helpline number: +44 (0)845 120 2918.
Website: www.laleche.org.uk; e-mail: enquiries@laleche.org.uk
For publications, LLL Books at above address, tel: +44 (0)845 456 1866; e-mail: books@laleche.org.uk.
Their aim is to help mothers to breast-feed through mother-to-mother support, encouragement, information and education; plus promote a better understanding of breast-feeding as an important element in the healthy development of the baby and mother.

Manic Depression Fellowship
Castle Works, 21 St George's Road, London SE1 6ES, UK
Tel: +44 0845 634 0540; fax: +44 (0)20 7793 2639
Website: www.mdf.org.uk; e-mail: mdf@mdf.org.uk
This charity has a national network of support groups and runs self-management training courses.

Marcé Society
PO Box 30853, London W12 OXG, UK
Website: www.marcesociety.com; e-mail: info@marcesociety.com
An international society for the understanding, prevention and treatment of mental illness related to child-bearing.

Maternity Alliance
Third Floor West, 2–6 Northburgh Street, London EC1V 0AY, UK
Tel: +44 (0)20 7490 7639; fax: +44 (0)20 7014 1350; information line: +44 (0)20 7490 7638
Website: www.maternityalliance.org.uk; e-mail: info@maternityalliance.org.uk
This gives information about all aspects of pregnancy and new parenthood. It also gives advice and has a factsheet on work rights and welfare benefits for women with PND.

Meet-A-Mum-Association (MAMA)
7 Southcourt Road, Linslade, Leighton Buzzard, Bedfordshire LU7 2QF, UK
Tel: +44 (0)1525 217 064; fax: +44 (0)20 8239 1153; postnatal depression helpline +44 0845 120 3746 (Monday to Friday 7 p.m.–10 p.m.)
Website: www.mama.co.uk; e-mail: meet-a-mum.assoc@btinternet.com
This association provides friendship and support to mothers and mothers-to-be, lonely or isolated, after the birth of a baby or moving to a new area. There are self-help groups for mothers with small children and specific help and support to women suffering from postnatal depression. There is a helpline and plenty of links and information.

Mind
15–19 Broadway, London E15 4BQ, UK
Tel: +44 (0)20 8519 2122; fax: +44 (0)20 8522 1725; Mind infoline: +44 (0)845 766 0163
Website: www.mind.org.uk; e-mail: contact@mind.org.uk
A UK-based mental health charity which publishes and sells a number of useful publications. Local Mind associations offer many services, including advocacy, crisis helplines, counselling, befriending, supported housing, employment, drop-in centres and training schemes, around the country.

Miscarriage Association
c/o Clayton Hospital, Northgate, Wakefield, West Yorkshire WF1 3JS, UK
Helpline: +44 (0)1924 200799; Scottish helpline: +44 (0)131 334 8883; fax: +44 (0)1924 298834
Website: www.miscarriageassociation.org.uk; e-mail: info@miscarriageassociation.org.uk

They provide support, give information, promote awareness and are working for better care.

Mothers for Mothers Post-Natal Depression Support Group
PO Box 1292, Bristol BS99 2FP, UK
Helpline: +44 (0)117 975 6006
Website: www.mothersformothers.fsnet.co.uk; e-mail: support@mothers formothers.fsnet.co.uk
A charity with funding for mothers in the Bristol, South Gloucestershire and Bath & North East Somerset areas only. However there are useful sources of information and links.

Mothersbliss
Mothersbliss Ltd, PO Box 240, Loughton, Essex IG10 1ZB, UK
Tel: +44 (0)20 8925 6150
Website: www.mothersbliss.com/; e-mail: getintouch@mothersbliss.com
A website for advice, guidance and help in selecting the correct products for yourself and your baby if you are planning a family, are pregnant now, or have a young family.

Mothers 35 plus
Website: www.mothers35plus.co.uk
Useful information and links in general for older mums.

Motherwise
Sue Wentworth-Sheilds MSc MInstD FRSA, Braygate House, North Somercotes, Lincolnshire LN11 7PS, UK
Tel: +44 (0)1507 358848
Website: www.motherwise.co.uk; e-mail: news@motherwise.co.uk
A website with over 100 pages of fun and information for every mum and every situation – 'celebrating the diversity of motherhood'. There are discussion forums too and links to absolutely loads of things both fun and educational.

Mumsnet
Website: www.mumsnet.com; e-mail: contactus@mumsnet.com
Mumsnet is an on-line network of parents pooling their knowledge on everything from how to get a baby to sleep through the night to the best places to go on holiday with a five-year-old. There are useful discussion areas on many topics.

National Childbirth Trust
Alexandra House, Oldham Terrace, Acton, London W3 6NH, UK
Tel: +44 (0)870 770 3236; enquiry line: +44 (0)870 444 8707;

membership line: +44 (0)870 990 8040; breast-feeding line: +44 (0)870 444 8708; fax: +44 (0)870 770 3237
Website: www.nctpregnancyandbabycare.com; e-mail: enquiries@national-childbirth-trust.co.uk
The Trust aims to help all parents enjoy an experience of pregnancy, birth and early parenthood which enriches their lives and gives them confidence in being a parent. They have a network of local branches concerned with antenatal and postnatal support through a range of antenatal classes, help-lines and social and educational events. They offer supportive groups to women before and after birth, and groups for depressed mothers. The National Childbirth Trust provides leaflets, books and videos on all aspects of parenting including PND. The NCT has a new book on PND available from NCT Maternity Sales (+44 (0)870 112 1120).

National Electronic Library for Mental Health (NeLMH)
Website: www.nelmh.org
This specialist library sits within the National Electronic Library for Health and aims to provide access to the best available evidence to answer your mental health questions. There are many links to NHS facilities.

National Health and Medical Research Council (Australia)
Website: www.nhmrc.gov.au/publications/synopses/wh29syn.htm; general enquiry: nhmrc.publications@nhmrc.gov.au
Details can be found here of an information paper *Postnatal Depression: a systematic review of published scientific literature to 1999*. It documents current multidisciplinary research results in the areas of prevalence, clinical presentation, course, assessment, treatment and prevention of post-natal depression. To support the information paper, NHMRC has also prepared a consumer guide, *Postnatal Depression: not just the baby blues*, to provide parents with advice and support on postnatal depression, describes symptoms and details how to find professional help and contact support groups Australia wide.

National NEWPIN
Sutherland House, 35 Sutherland Square, Walworth, London SE17 3EE, UK
Tel: +44 (0)20 7358 5900; fax: +44 (0)20 7701 2660
Website: www.newpin.org.uk; e-mail: info@newpin.org.uk
NEWPIN works with parents and other primary carers of children who are in need of support in their role as parents by offering attachment and befriending, individual counselling and group therapy for parents and play therapy for children. They have centres around London, in Chesterfield and in Northern Ireland.

One Parent Families
255 Kentish Town Road, London NW5 2LX, UK
Tel: +44 (0)20 7428 5400; fax: +44 (0)20 7482 4851; helpline : +44 (0)800 018 5026 (Monday to Friday 9 a.m.–5 p.m.); fax: +44 (0)20 7482 4851
Website: www.oneparentfamilies.org.uk; e-mail: info@oneparentfamilies.org.uk
One Parent Families represents lone parents and their children in England and Wales. It aims to promote the welfare of lone parents and their children and to overcome the poverty, isolation and social exclusion which so many face. They offer parents the means to help themselves and their families by providing information and advice, working with communities, and by developing new solutions to meet changing needs.

Online PPD Support Group
Tonya Rosenberg, PO Box 611, Issaquah, WA 98027-0023, USA
Website: www.ppdsupportpage.com/; e-mail: tonya@ppdsupportpage.com
This is a site run by women who have suffered from postnatal illness. It is based in the US but has useful links and resources.

Pacific Post Partum Support Society
104–1416 Commercial Drive, Vancouver BC V5L 3X9 CANADA
Tel: +1 604 255 7999; fax: +1 604 255 7588
Website: www.postpartum.org
The Pacific Post Partum Support Society (PPPSS) is a non-profit society which provides support to women and families experiencing depression or anxiety related to the birth or adoption of a baby. They also provide training and information for professionals, as well as community education on postpartum depression.

PaNDa
Post and Ante Natal Depression Association, Inc., 270 Church Street, Richmond, Victoria 3121, Australia
PaNDa administration and support line: +61 (0)2 9428 4600; fax: +61 (0)3 9428 2400; (office hours are 9.30 a.m.–4.30 p.m., Monday to Thursday)
Website: www.panda.org.au/; e-mail: panda@vicnet.net.au
This is an Australian association which aims to support and inform women, and their families, who are affected by post- and antenatal mood disorders, as well as educating healthcare professionals and the wider community. There are information pages and links to other sources of support in addition to locally based events.

Parents Place
Website: www.parentsplace.com/pregnancy; this is part of www.iVillage.com
Parents Place is a US website for all matters concerning pregnancy, birth and family. There are links to information and discussion about postpartum (postnatal) issues.

Pendulum
Website: www.pendulum.org
Pendulum Resources is the web presence of the Pendulum e-mail list, an on-line support group for manic-depressives. It is an extensive site and contains a lot of useful information.

PNDSA (Post-Natal Depression Support Association of South Africa)
Website: www.pndsa.co.za/; e-mail secretary: colleen@pndsa.co.za
PNDSA is a non-profit-making association started by a group of health professionals and women who have recovered from postnatal depression. They are dedicated to supporting other women who may be going through the same experience and to making it easier for them to find help. There are plenty of informative pages.

PND Training
Website: www.pndtraining.co.uk; e-mail: info@pndtraining.co.uk
A site with information about training for health professionals in the detection and treatment of PND.

Post-partum-depression.com
NCERx LLC, 5928 Geiger St, Carlsbad, CA 92008, USA
Tel: +1 (800) 549 3904
Website: www.post-partum-depression.com; e-mail: webmaster@e-health-questions.info
A healthcare site offering information on symptoms and treatment and a discussion forum.

Postpartum Support International
Website: www.postpartum.net/
An American site full of tips, resources and information plus contacts within the US and worldwide. The 'moms and family page' is especially useful. Likewise, their link to www.postpartumdads.org is a useful site which addresses the needs of men whose wife/partner suffers from PPD.

Pregnancy and Birth with Robin Elise Weiss
Website: www.pregnancy.about.com
A USA site with advice on all aspects of pregnancy and birth with specific advice on postpartum (postnatal) issues.

Raising Kids

General enquiries: +44 (0)20 8883 8621

Website: www.raisingkids.co.uk/

A parenting resource for anyone raising kids. There are items about every topic you can think of with links for resources and discussion forums. Its aim is 'to offer support, information and friendship to everyone who's raising kids – whatever your circumstances or income'.

Relate

Herbert Gray College, Little Church Street, Rugby, Warwickshire CV21 3AP, UK

Relateline tel: +44 (0)845 130 4010 (Monday to Friday, 9.30 a.m.–4.30 p.m.); switchboard: +44 (0)845 456 1310

Website: www.relate.org.uk; e-mail: enquiries@relate.org.uk

A source of information and advice about relationships and counselling. They offer courses for new parents.

Royal College of Psychiatrists

17 Belgrave Square, London SW1X 8PG, UK

Tel: +44 (0)20 7235 2351; fax: +44 (0)20 7245 1231

Website: www.rcpsych.ac.uk; e-mail: rcpsych@rcpsych.ac.uk

Articles and links to sources of information and help with PND.

Samaritans

The Upper Mill, Kingston Road, Ewell, Surrey, KT17 2AF, UK

Tel: +44 (0)20 8394 8300; fax: +44 (0)20 8394 8301

Website: www.samaritans.org; e-mail: admin@samaritans.org (for administration details)

The Samaritans offer a 24-hour confidential, emotional support line. National: +44 (0)845 790 9090 (UK); Republic of Ireland: +353 1850 60 90 90.

For potential callers there are additional contacts by e-mail: jo@samaritans.org or write to: Chris, PO Box 90, Stirling, Stirlingshire FK8 2SA, UK.

Samaritans is a registered charity based in the UK and Republic of Ireland that provides confidential emotional support to any person who is suicidal or despairing. It also increases public awareness of issues around suicide and depression.

SANE

SANE, 1st Floor, Cityside House, 40 Adler Street, London E1 1EE, UK

Tel: +44 (0)20 7375 1002; Saneline: +44 (0)845 767 8000 (12 noon–2 a.m.)

Website: www.sane.org.uk; e-mail: london@sane.org.uk (for admin queries)

SANE has three main objectives:

1 To raise awareness and respect for people with mental illness and their families, improve education and training, and secure better services.
2 To initiate and fund research into the causes of serious mental illness through the Prince of Wales International Centre for SANE Research.
3 To provide information and emotional support to those experiencing mental health problems, their families and carers through Saneline.

Sheila Kitzinger website
Website: www.sheilakitzinger.com; e-mail: tess@sheilakitzinger.com
Here you can explore aspects of birth, drawing on things that author Sheila has learned from women around the world and her research as a social anthropologist into women's experiences of pregnancy, birth and breast-feeding. Sheila runs a Birth Crisis Network, a phone service for women who need to talk about traumatic birth experiences with some one who understands and listens reflectively. The number is her own phone number: +44 (0)1865 300 266 and she can often put callers in touch with someone who has been to one of her workshops and who is nearer them.

Siobhan Curham's website
Website: www.geocities.com/anteandpostnataldepression; e-mail: anteand postnataldepression@yahoo.co.uk
This site, written by a sufferer, offers advice and information on ante- and postnatal depression.

Sure Start
Sure Start Unit, Department for Education and Skills and Department for Work and Pensions, Level 2, Caxton House, Tothill Street, London SW1H 9NA, UK
Public Enquiry Unit tel: +44 (0)870 000 2288
Website: www.surestart.gov.uk; e-mail: info.surestart@dfes.gsi.gov.uk
Sure Start is the Government's programme to deliver the best start in life for every child by bringing together early education, child care, health and family support. There are a number of programmes around the country, some which offer specific support for PND.

TABS – Trauma And Birth Stress – New Zealand
P O Box 18002, Glen Innes, Auckland, New Zealand
Tel: +64 (0)8324 8227
Website: www.tabs.org.nz; e-mail: sue@tabs.org.nz.
TABS (Trauma And Birth Stress) originated in New Zealand. It is a chari-table trust formed by a support group of mothers who have in common

stressful and traumatic pregnancies or births that affected their lives negatively for months or years afterwards. They formed TABS because of the need to make post traumatic stress disorder (PTSD) known as a form of mental illness that can happen following childbirth, but that is quite distinct from the baby blues, postnatal depression (post partum depression) and postnatal psychosis.

Threshold Women's Mental Health Infoline
Threshold Women's Mental Health Initiative, 14 St George's Place, Brighton, East Sussex BN1 4GB, UK
Tel: +44 (0)1273 626444 (Monday to Thursday, 2 p.m.–4.30 p.m.; Monday & Wednesday, 10 a.m.–12 p.m. There is a 24-hour answerphone outside opening hours.)
Website: www.thresholdwomen.org.uk; e-mail: thrwomen@gxn.co.uk
They provide details of local and national services throughout the UK; wide-ranging information about mental health issues; a series of factsheets on women and mental health plus emotional support for women seeking information. They help women experiencing mental health difficulties and those experiencing emotional distress; and their carers, families, friends and partners and workers supporting women with mental health issues.

United Kingdom Council for Psychotherapy
167–169 Great Portland Street, London W1W 5P, UK
Tel: +44 (0)20 7436 3002; fax: +44 (0)20 7436 3013
Website: www.psychotherapy.org.uk; e-mail: ukcp@psychotherapy.org.uk
The main organisation for psychotherapy in the UK. Regional lists of psychotherapists are available free of charge.

UK Parents
Website: www.ukparents.co.uk
A parenting resource with lots of information and expert advice on preconception, pregnancy, labour and birth, babies and toddlers. Many discussion forums are available, including one for PND.

Unplanned Pregnancies
Website: unplannedpregnancies.co.uk; e-mail: guinness_maiden@hotmail.com
This site offers information on ante- and postnatal depression, as well as exploring your choices if you have an unplanned pregnancy.

Veritee Reed Hall's website
Website: www.pni.org.uk; forum: veritee.proboards7.com/
A UK website offering PND support and information. The discussion forum is very active.

WellMother

Website: www.wellmother.com; e-mail: smisri@wellmother.com

WellMother.com is an on-line resource for women and their families, designed to offer support and resources on a number of issues related to the emotional challenges of the reproductive cycle, including postnatal. There is a comprehensive links page for both Canadian and international websites, books and resources.

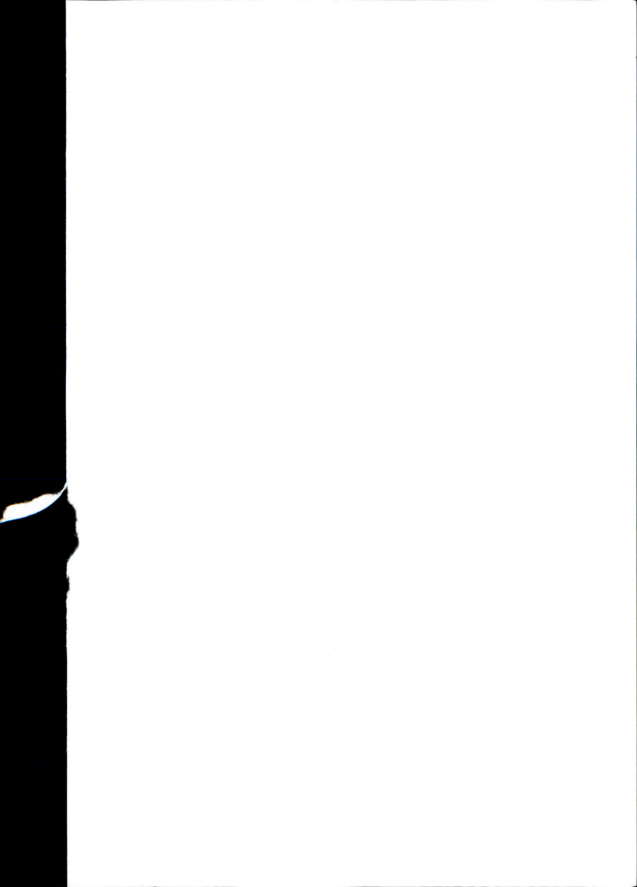

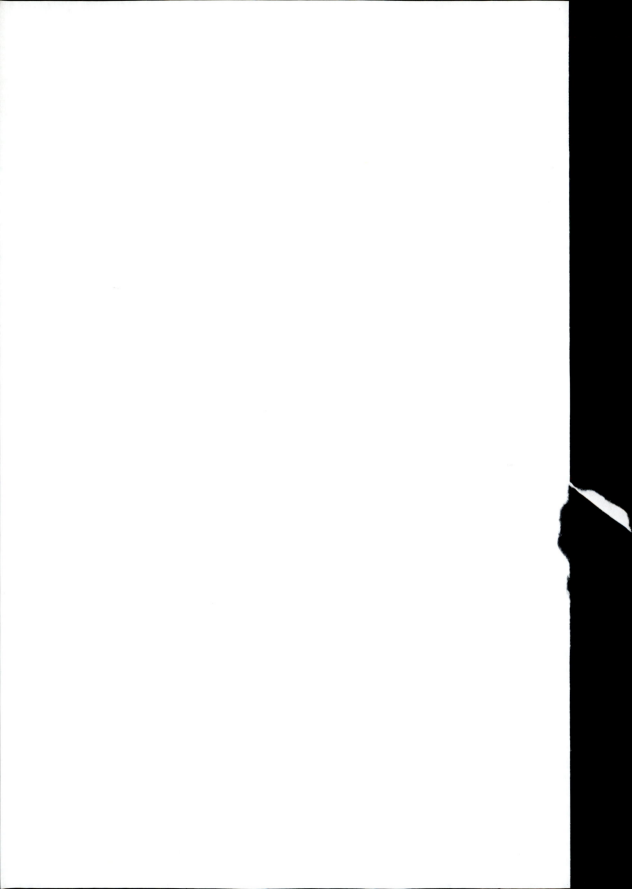